C000301337

Dr Alan Howard is an acknowledged autł
disease from a nutritional point of view. N⟨
of Downing College, University of Camł
Cambridge University for over 50 yea
Department of Medicine and the Dunn
research in the Department of Pathology, ᵣ.. ⌐ᵣ
of Medicine on Obesity research. He founded and supported from 1990 to 1997
the COAG Laboratory at Papworth Hospital, Cambridge – one of the leading
heart hospitals in the UK, which specialised in nutritional aspects of coronary
heart disease.

He has published over 250 original articles in the medical literature and has
authored and edited eight books. He was founder of the International Journal
of Obesity together with Dr George Bray, of the University of California, Los
Angeles, and edited the proceedings of the First International Congress on
Obesity in London.

He was founder member and first secretary of the European Atherosclerosis
Society and organised their first International Congress in Athens .

He is the inventor of the Cambridge Diet, a very low calorie diet (VLCD),
which has been used world-wide for the treatment of obesity since 1980. It is
now available in 25 countries, not only as a VLCD, but also as the nutritional
foundation of a range of weight management programmes at different calorific
levels.

In 1982 he established the Howard Foundation, a charitable Foundation
which has donated  $6 million for the Howard Building, at Downing College,
Cambridge University. In 2000 he was awarded a Wilkins Fellowship by the
college in recognition of his major contributions.

The Foundation receives its income from the companies owned by Howard
Foundation Holdings of which he is chairman. Over the last 10 years, through
the work of Dr Howard, the Foundation has invested in research into the use
of creatine, red wine polyphenols, and certain carotenoids preventing age-
related macular degeneration, the major cause of blindness in the elderly.

In 1996 Dr Howard was honoured by the award of an Honorary Doctorate
at the University of Ulster in Northern Ireland, in recognition of his
establishment of the Howard Foundation Chair of Human Nutrition and has
recently been made a visiting Professor there.

In 2001, the Duke of Edinburgh, Chancellor of Cambridge University,
invested Dr Howard as a Companion of the of the Guild of Cambridge
Benefactors.

The first edition of this book, published by Jonathan Cape Limited in 1985, received the following reviews:

*'Tells the whole story in layman's language'*

Sunday Times

*'A unique diet breakthrough'*

Southport Visitor

*'A dieting revolution'*

Bournemouth Evening Echo

*'The diet that really does work wonders'*

News of the World

*'A diet that peels the pounds off fast'*

Glasgow Herald

*'Summers' newest guru has found the fastest, most healthy way to lose weight'*

Daily Express

# The Cambridge Diet

*TRIED, TESTED & TRUSTED*
**Cambridge**
*WORLDWIDE*

## Dr Alan N Howard

## Twentieth Anniversary Edition

Cambridge Manufacturing Company Limited

**To Ian McLean Baird, MD, FRCP**

THE CAMBRIDGE DIET

Originally published in Great Britain by Jonathan Cape Ltd.

**PRINTING HISTORY**
Jonathan Cape edition published 1985
Corgi edition published 1986
Corgi edition reprinted 1986 (four times)
Corgi edition reprinted 1987 (twice)

Cambridge 20th Anniversary edition published 2004

This book is set in 10/11.5 Palatino

Published by Cambridge Manufacturing Company Limited
Stafford House, Brakey Road
Corby, Northants, NN17 1LU
ISBN 0-9546557-0-2
Printed and bound in Great Britain by
Page Bros, Norwich

# Contents

# Notes

## Medical Precautions

Cambridge Health and Weight Plan recommends that everyone planning to start a weight-loss programme should advise their doctor.

Medical supervision is particularly important when losing weight for the very elderly, for growing children and adolescents, or for those with heart and cardiovascular conditions, diabetes, gout, kidney disease, stroke, chronic infections, hypoglycaemia, or those who are under medical care for any other condition.

Within the United Kingdom, Cambridge offers a range of weight-loss programmes, from around 400 calories to 1500 calories per day. Although everyone may use Cambridge as a nutritional supplement, those with certain medical conditions – or on particular medications – may not be able to use a weight-loss programme. These conditions are fully discussed in Chapter 4.

The Cambridge Diet should not be used as the sole source of nutrition for more than four consecutive weeks unless under medical supervision.

## Cambridge around the world

This edition of "The Cambridge Diet" has been produced to co-incide with the twentieth anniversary of the launch in the United Kingdom. Consequently, the book is presented from the point of view of a typical dieter in the UK. However, Cambridge is available in more than 20 countries around the world, with only minor changes to flavours, ingredients and the method of distribution in order to meet local regulations.

The Cambridge Diet currently available in the United States under that name is not the same, and is not the same product that was launched as The Cambridge Diet in the USA in 1980.

# Foreword to the 1985 Edition

*Sir John Butterfield, MD, FRCP (1920– 2000)*

*(Then Regius Professor of Physic, Cambridge University)*

I have known Alan Howard for twenty years as a very energetic biochemist and nutritionist. We first became acquainted through our shared research interests. He was particularly concerned about obese people, and at that time I and my colleagues at Guy's Hospital, in London, were looking into the adult onset of diabetes in patients who are usually overweight. For example, why would glucose not move from the blood of ordinary fat people into their muscles (unless they exercised) as it did in thin people? In a way we were finding that almost all fat people were partially diabetic.

Alan Howard's approach to all this was more straightforward, more practical and much more directly concerned with doing something about the obesity. Quite simply, he wanted to find out the best way to help people become thin, and so he set to work along these lines in the Department of Medicine at Cambridge.

Early on, he was interested in what he called the 'Cambridge Loaf', from which much of the carbohydrate had been extracted before the flour was used to make the dough. Then he began to see that it was important not only to provide a low calorie diet but one which also ensured that the dieter would not go without vitamins, minerals or trace elements. He wanted a diet which, if possible, would not turn the body's defences to retaining water and so hinder weight loss. In due course, his clinical colleagues joined in the work and it became clear that their new formula, based on fortified skimmed milk powder, could help people lose weight in a satisfactory way. And it was soon appreciated that the diet had to be so tasty that people really looked forward to taking it, rather than dreading it.

This is the background to the story which Alan Howard has set out in his book. Of course, there have been ups and downs in his adventures, while he searched for an ideal weight reducing diet. He faced problems trying to find a British firm to follow his lead, and then ran into difficulties with some critical members of the medical profession in the USA. Pioneers in these things never have an easy or instant success, especially in a field like weight reduction. Yet Alan's personal sense of purpose, of urgency, and his genuine concern for overweight people, individuals who need his skills and ideas and his persuasion in order to help themselves, all come over strongly in these pages.

Here then is the story of an exceptional scientist, who has shown perseverance in this basic research work and persistence in his efforts to develop his ideas with a view to helping not only a very large number of overweight people but, maybe soon, other categories of patients as well. I will be surprised if the reader of this fascinating book is not gripped by its account of his efforts so far, and its presentation of ideas he is developing for the future.

# Preface to Twentieth Anniversary Edition

The Cambridge Diet arose out of more than eight years of research and development at the University of Cambridge and the West Middlesex and Addenbrookes Hospitals in the UK. The original formula – which contained only 330 kilocalories (kcal) – was otherwise complete in all essential nutrients. Subsequently, the formula has been developed and improved to form the basis for a number of weight management programmes ranging from just over 400 kcal to 1500 kcal per day. At the lower end of this scale, dieters use Cambridge as 'the sole source' of nutrition, with substantial weight losses achieved with absolute safety. At the higher calorie levels, Cambridge is used as a nutritional foundation together with selected conventional food to promote more gradual weight loss, weight stabilisation and long-term weight maintenance.

The Cambridge Diet was originally introduced in the Spring of 1980 in the United States, which was followed by a UK launch in 1984. Since then, it has spread around the world, across Europe and into Asia, the Middle East and South America, so that it is now available in more than twenty countries.

The Diet is available through a variety of outlets often using distributors – or 'Cambridge Counsellors', who themselves have benefited from using Cambridge and want to help others do the same – but also, in some countries, through health professionals, health and beauty clinics, health food stores and pharmacies. Common to all is the provision of information, advice and support for the dieter. Through the past twenty years of development and growth, it is estimated that more than 20 million people worldwide have used Cambridge successfully to manage their weight, and continuing research has provided evidence that the programmes work.

Despite obvious success, in its early days the Diet attracted controversy and criticism – often the case with a new and exciting development. At first it was maintained that the formulation of the Diet was contrary to current nutritional principles, despite having a balance of all nutrients. Later on experts admitted the Diet was effective but felt it should only be used under supervision in specialised clinics and university medical schools.

The reality in the world today, however, is quite different. Thousands of general practitioners found that their patients experienced significant weight losses, with very minor or no side effects, and in many countries even the Very Low Calorie Diet programme is freely available within the community as well as in primary, secondary and occupational health care. In fact, many people have managed their weight with Cambridge and have changed their lives for the better! I have included a number of their stories in this book. All the people interviewed have given permission for their names to be used.

The twentieth anniversary of the launch of the Cambridge Diet in the UK is an ideal opportunity to up-date this book, to explain how and why Cambridge programmes are effective, and to help dispel many of the misconceptions that have arisen about it.

*Alan Howard*
*Cambridge, 2004*


For further information about the availability of the diet, please contact
    Cambridge Health and Weight Plan,
    Stafford House, Brakey Road
    Corby, Northants, NN17 1LU
or visit the website at www.cambridge-diet.com

# Acknowledgements

When I originally wrote "The Cambridge Diet" in 1985, there were many people who helped and to whom I owed grateful thanks. Among them were Eleanor Harnish from Norman, Oklahoma, Mary Miller and Rita Steffensen as well as members of my family and others who read the manuscript and made valuable suggestions. This 20th Anniversary edition has been brought up to date with the invaluable help of Alan Harris and Eileen Skinner, who have attempted to retain the spirit of my original text, whilst acknowledging how Cambridge is used throughout the world today.

Writing this book also gives me the opportunity to thank all those who participated in the development and clinical trials of the Cambridge Diet. Among the foremost of these is Dr Ian McLean Baird, to whom this book is dedicated and without whom the work could never have been accomplished; Professor Sir John A.H. Butterfield, head of the Clinical School, University of Cambridge, for his interest and moral support; Professor Ivor Mills for allowing the work to take place in his department and for constant encouragement. Among the doctors who supervised the Obesity Clinic at Addenbrooke's Hospital were Andrew Grant, Ray Moore, Russell Cook, Steve Olczak, John Marks, Andrew Brooks and Huw Alban Davies. Technical assistance was given by Michael and Betty Brown, Aileen Bright, and Shashi Rattan. At the West Middlesex Hospital, the doctors included Ray Parsons and ER Littlewood. The project could never have succeeded without the untiring devotion of Joan Fowler, who was in charge of the day-to-day handling of the inpatients at the West Middlesex Hospital. On the commercial side, I am especially indebted to Dennis Jones, without whose help the Diet certainly would never have been made accessible to the public; also to Jack, Eileen and Vaughn Feather, of Monterey, California, who had the foresight to see its great potential.

# Part One - The Cambridge Plan

# The Weight Problem 1

## Introduction

Overweight and obesity are not new problems, and they are not local problems. In a recent technical report, the World Health Organisation drew attention to the extent of the problem of obesity:

*"... obesity is one of today's most blatantly visible – yet most neglected – public health problems. Paradoxically coexisting with undernutrition, an escalating global epidemic of overweight and obesity – "globesity" – is taking over many parts of the world. If immediate action is not taken, millions will suffer from an array of serious health disorders.*

*"Obesity is a complex condition, one with serious social and psychological dimensions, that affects virtually all age and socioeconomic groups and threatens to overwhelm both developed and developing countries. In 1995, there were an estimated 200 million obese adults worldwide and another 18 million under-five children classified as overweight. As of 2000, the number of obese adults has increased to over 300 million. Contrary to conventional wisdom, the obesity epidemic is not restricted to industrialized societies; in developing countries, it is estimated that over 115 million people suffer from obesity-related problems."*

Within the United Kingdom, the National Audit Office (NAO) produced an important report: "Tackling Obesity in England" in 2001. In their report, the NAO showed that in 1998, nearly a fifth of all adults were obese, whilst more than half the women – and two-thirds of the men – were at least overweight.

## Where Overweight Starts

Most people have an image of the weight and shape they would like to be. Sometimes, this is realistic and healthy; sometimes it isn't and is driven by media or peer pressure. But, achieving a 'healthy' weight has never been easy and in the twenty-first century has become even harder.

We watch more television, play more video games or surf the internet; we watch rather than play sport; we eat and drink out more than we used to – often choosing high-fat, high sugar and high salt options.

It isn't just a matter of cosmetic vanity. Insurance companies have realised for many years that they are likely to have to pay out more on life assurance policies on overweight or obese customers. Overweight – or pre-obesity – and obesity itself are serious health issues for individuals, healthcare providers and governments.

> ## The higher the weight, the greater the risk, in a very dramatic way.

## Increased Health Risks

When the body is forced into carrying extra weight, it puts an additional burden on every part of the system. The heart has to work harder, as do the muscles and lungs. Obesity is linked closely to high blood pressure, which puts the individual at risk of a stroke. The good news here is that as weight is lost, blood pressure tends to go down. So in this area, at least, the damage can be reversed.

There's an association with overweight and a whole raft of heart conditions. Obese patients develop diabetes more often and register more deaths from a certain list of cancers – colorectal and prostrate in men and cervical, ovarian, breast and gallbladder in women. Gallstones and liver diseases are linked with overweight as are gout, hernias and varicose veins.

As if all this wasn't bad enough, warm, sweaty recesses between folds of skin are ideal breeding grounds for microbes that lead to skin disorders. And the obese are even less likely to have a good night's sleep!

Today, health professionals and other interested people use a reliable measure of overweight and risk: the body mass index.

## Body Mass Index (BMI)

BMI is essentially the ratio between your weight and the square of your height, using metric measurements (see box, right).

$$BMI \quad \frac{weight\ (kg)}{height\ (m) \times height\ (m)}$$

For example, someone who is 5ft 11in (1.8m) tall, weighing 165lb (75kg) would have a BMI of 75/(1.8 x 1.8) = 75 / 3.24 = 23.

It has been generally agreed that between BMI 20 and BMI 25 is an acceptable healthy range in western populations. In South-East Asia, this 'acceptable' range lies between BMI 18 and BMI 23.

The reason for allowing a range of BMI values is because it would be unreasonable to expect a large boned, heavy set man to weigh the same as someone who was much slighter in build but the same height. So, this BMI 'normal' range provides plenty of scope for different frame structures. For example, the 1.8m tall person introduced earlier could weigh anywhere between 67kg and 83kg and still record a BMI of 20 to 25.

## Health Risks

| Classification | BMI | Risk | Waist |
|---|---|---|---|
| Underweight | below 20 | | |
| Healthy range | between 20-25 | Normal | over 37in (men) |
| Overweight | betweenn 25-30 | Increased | over 37in (men) |
| Obese | between 30 –40 | Moderate | over 40in (men) |
| Morbidly obese | greater than 40 | Very severe | |

Source:
Obesity: Preventing and Managing the Global Epidemic. Report of
World Health Organisation Consultation on Obesity. WHO 1998

## Target Weight

Finding out someone's BMI is easy, if the height and weight are known (see Appendix 2).

☐   do the long division !

☐   use a BMI chart

☐   use a BMI slide rule calculator

The end target weight should be below BMI 25 for medical reasons and within the range 20 to 25 for reasons of self-esteem and personal image. So, the target weight should be in the range 20 to 25 according to personal preference. Remember however, that if a dieter stops dieting at BMI 25, any weight regained places them in the overweight range.

Although there is no scientific evidence to support it, BMI 23 is a sensible value to aim for, being in the middle of the 'normal' range and having little or no risk to health. The number 23 is also useful because the BMI equation above can be re-organised to calculate a target weight:

height (metres) x height (metres) x BMI = target weight (kilograms)

Since the height, which is unlikely to change, is known and BMI value is known (23) the target weight can be calculated.

For example, someone who is 5ft 6in (1.67m), would have a Target of 23 x 1.67 x 1.67 = (141lb) 64kg

## A Growing Problem

Successive governments and other organisations around the world have produced reports giving advice on how to eat healthily. All have been accompanied by media articles, books and magazines full of scare stories about how fat we are. But, despite sound, sensible advice on healthy eating and lifestyle, despite shocking details of the prevalence of overweight, the situation is getting worse.

Because obesity has such a negative impact on health, its effects create a huge national economic burden as well. For example, did you know that in England alone in 1998, obesity accounted for nearly 18 million days off work? At the current rate of increase, these absent days could amount to 21 million by 2005, and over 25 million in 2010.

These are just the short-term effects. What about the longer-term? Obesity is a major factor in chronic life-threatening conditions such as heart disease, strokes, cancers and diabetes. Once again using figures and estimates from the NAO Report, we find that, in 1998, just over 40,000 years of working life were lost because of obesity and its effects. By 2005, this number of 'lost years of working life' could be more than 47,000, rising to a staggering 59,000 by the end of the decade if the NAO's predictions on the rise of obesity are correct.

So, obesity carries a huge cost – and not only in human terms. The NAO estimates that the total cost of obesity and its effects could reach over £3.5billion by 2010. In addition to the increased medical risks to the overweight, there are other burdens just as difficult to bear.

For example, many seriously overweight patients are being given an ultimatum by their doctors; lose the weight – or lose the operation. Surgeons are becoming more reluctant to operate on overweight people because it complicates every aspect of their work: the procedure itself; the anaesthesia; and the overall rate of healing. Faced with the prospect of not getting the operation they need, the patients are forced to do something about their weight.

In fact, from a health risk point of view, the graph begins to 'take off' at around BMI 30. Insurance actuaries have plotted the risk of premature death relative to weight. Let's say that the 20 – 25 BMI target range has an index of 100 – in other words it has a neutral effect on premature death; a BMI of 30 will increase your index to around 125 which means you have a 25% higher chance of premature death. At BMI 40, the index rockets to 280 – or almost tripling the risk of an early death; and this is a greater risk to health than smoking 20 cigarettes a day.

Leaving aside medical considerations, the overweight also suffer huge social and psychological pressures. Most people think that they are inferior to thin people; that they are undisciplined and permanently unhappy. Consequently, overweight people face discrimination at school and at work. And consequently many overweight people have very low self-esteem.

Any way you look at it, there are plenty of sound logical reasons for not being overweight.

# The Perfect Diet

*2*

Newspapers and magazines are full of articles about slimming. 'Lose 5lb (2kg) In Five Days' is the sort of headline frequently seen in our Sunday newspapers. It seems that very many people are obsessed with losing weight.

Dieting is by no means an easy undertaking. In fact it is extremely difficult. Mark Twain's remark about smoking – 'It's easy to give up, I've done it many times' – is equally true of slimming.

There are innumerable systems of dieting in existence – someone even published an encyclopedia which listed over 200 diets. Those people who follow any one of these diets will almost certainly lose some weight. The first 5lb (2kg) will fall off easily – because most of it is water – but what then?

People approach dieting in different ways, but a number of generalizations can be made. When it comes to giving up eating, many of us are only willing to make sacrifices for a short time. We like food; it is very pleasurable. On the other hand, dieting is inconvenient; it interferes with parties, business lunches, holidays, and makes us feel like social outcasts.

So, for many people, the perfect diet should guarantee rapid loss of weight, so that the resumption of eating whatever is considered to be 'Real Food' may begin as soon as possible. For others, a more gradual approach to weight loss will suit their lifestyle better.

## Approaches to Losing Weight

*Consume fewer calories than your body uses.*

This is the only way to lose weight. You can add to this rule that exercise tones up your body and provides other health benefits. But every diet in the world boils down to this simple reality. The difference between them is not what they do for you – but HOW they work.

Anyone who has been on a diet knows the most important thing there is to know about diets: there are no magic solutions to losing weight. The weight maintenance formula is very simple and it can be written in a number of ways (see box overleaf):

## Weight Loss Equation

energy expended **more than** calories taken in **means** weight loss

energy expended **equals** calories taken in **means** weight balance

energy expended **less than** calories taken in **means** weight gain

So, what can you do to lose weight? There are only five different methods:

☐ you can reduce the amount of food you eat

☐ you can change your eating behaviour

☐ you can increase your activity level and exercise more

☐ you can count calories

☐ you can use a very low-calorie diet

## Reducing food consumption

For some people, a little moderation is all they need to bring their weight back to the desired level. The closer they are to their target weight, the more effective this approach will be. For anyone but the mildly overweight, though, the effectiveness of moderation is slight. Often the underlying cause of initial weight gain was a lack of willpower and motivation, so it's unlikely that these qualities will suddenly appear in sufficient strength to achieve the desired target.

There's also the influence of the body's metabolic rate – or the rate at which the body burns energy to go about its daily task. As the body loses weight, the metabolic rate will automatically drop slightly – which means that the body is now burning calories at a lower rate. To carry on losing weight, you have to reduce consumption even more. In other words, moderation can easily be self defeating.

## Changing Eating Behaviour

Except in a few, very specific cases, overweight is usually caused by deep-rooted behaviour from the past, or current lifestyle stresses. Sometimes, this is due to a love of food, but there are plenty of other reasons: a wish to blot out depression or a way of getting over worry and stress for example.

But overweight or obese people seem to eat in a quite different way to others. They eat more quickly, take larger mouthfuls, chew less and drink much more with their food. In other words, they are probably not eating to satisfy hunger, but responding to other cues – such as the time of day or watching television. Research has shown that people can be helped by behaviour counselling, but at a very high cost in terms of professional involvement.

## Increasing Activity Levels

The need for regular exercise is the central theme for the "natural is best" approach. But, although it has many other important benefits, exercise will not account for very much weight loss if used in isolation. Very few people will be willing to set aside time for a regular exercise routine, and others simply shy away at the mention of the word "exercise". For most people, therefore, compliance is a problem. In fact, for the seriously overweight, exercise is not always physically possible – or for that matter immediately recommended – partly due to the exertion of shifting their extra bulk but also because of the risk of damage to joints. At Cambridge, we prefer to talk about activity levels rather than exercise, and recommend taking advantage of natural activities – such as a walk to the shops, rather than using the car.

Another important issue is that, for most normal activities, the additional energy expended is a relatively small proportion of the body's daily energy needs. So, although increased activity will improve your cardio-vascular performance and respiratory system, tone your muscles and improve your overall feeling of well being, it will not burn away many of those extra pounds. For example, a 1995 study estimated that weight lost by exercise alone was in the order of 100g a week. To lose 1kg of fat you need to use up 7,700kcal, and although the rate at which calories are burned depends on body weight, a person weighing 135lb (61kg) could expend 360 calories in a one-hour bike ride; he or she would need to pedal for over 21 hours to burn off that kilogram! Exercise is discussed further in Chapter 7.

## Counting Calories

On "average", women need to consume around 2000 kcal a day (2500 for men) to maintain a healthy weight. So the conventional carbohydrate/fat restricted diet would limit the intake to under 1500kcal (men = 2000kcal). At this level, providing the diet is drawn from a wide variety of foods, it is unlikely that there would be a significant lack of vitamins and minerals. However, it becomes very difficult to ensure that the Recommended Daily Allowance (RDA) of vitamins and minerals is being met once the diet drops below 1200kcal.

The other complication of the 'counting calories' approach is the actual counting process. Even with the help of a trained dietician, it is very difficult to be sure of the real calorie content of a meal, and it gets even worse if we do the counting ourselves. At best, counting calories with the use of tables is nothing more than a good guess. In reality, studies show that the figures are likely to be widely inaccurate, because not only is there the complication of having to weigh everything, most people are notoriously inaccurate when it comes to recording what they eat. Even the odd mint to freshen your breath or the extra half spoon of cream accounts for some additional calories. In the worse case scenario, some dieters either tell fibs or delude themselves about what they have consumed.

Counting calories has to be the most tedious and soul destroying job around. No wonder people get fed up with this approach. Every time they want to eat, out comes the log book, calorie tables and weight scales. It's enough to try the patience of a saint.

## Very Low Calorie Diets

With so many factors complicating conventional dieting, it is no wonder that many people experience poor results. While theoretically a diet of 1500 kcal or less should force the body to lose weight, hitting that level in a way that is both practical and enjoyable is not always achievable.

So, many years ago, the search was on for an effective alternative. Initially, a zero calorie diet attracted the attention of researchers. To the layman the prospect of no calories whatsoever seems bizarre, but given careful supervision by trained medical specialists in hospital conditions, this approach was extremely effective on a number of grossly obese patients. The results were dramatic but far from practical. Without careful supervision the technique would be very dangerous, so a zero calorie diet is not a realistic option for the general public.

But as long ago as the 1920s, people were trying minimal calorie diets as a means of achieving rapid weight loss without harmful side effects. Eventually, commercial diets began to appear on the market, and were known as very low calorie diets (VLCD).

## Cambridge Diet Programmes Explained

So what constitutes the perfect diet? My thinking is shown in the box below.

---

### The Perfect Diet

- ☐  is easy to use
- ☐  is relatively inexpensive
- ☐  has nutritional assurance
- ☐  is healthy
- ☐  has few side effects
- ☐  is fundamentally safe
- ☐  produces excellent weight-loss
- ☐  in the desired time-scale

For many people, this latter point means within a few weeks or, at the most, two or three months, to obtain their ideal body weight.

---

I believe that Cambridge programmes fulfil all the requirements of a 'perfect' diet.

The Cambridge Diet is a nutritionally complete formula food which is available in a range of weight-loss programmes. The diet is very easy and pleasant to take and comes in a number of different guises – as individual meals in sachets of powder which are mixed with water to produce soups and milkshakes; as ready-mixed Tetra Briks; and as chocolate-covered meal bars. Cambridge is available in a number of flavours, each representing a 'meal' of about 137 kcal*.

The weight-loss programmes start at just over 400 kilocalories (kcal) per day and, with the addition of selected conventional foods, they rise to 1500 kcal per day. An overweight person following the diet uses his or her body fat as fuel – just like a camel. So long as there is body fat available to provide energy the dieter will lose weight safely and surely! Moreover, they have the assurance that Cambridge will provide all the essential nutrients that the body needs whilst they are dieting.

*  Flavour ranges and calorific content may vary from country to country

Within the United Kingdom, Cambridge is sold through 'Cambridge Counsellors'. Counsellors have usually benefited previously by losing weight themselves, or having used the diet as a nutritional supplement. Their main purpose is to inspire others to emulate their own weight management success, to help ensure that the diet is used correctly, to offer support and encouragement and to answer questions. Although Cambridge Counsellors are trained and accredited by the Company, they are independent business people in their own right. (Cambridge Counsellors – and the distribution methods used in other parts of the world – are discussed further in Chapter 5.)

## The Programmes

(see the 'Steps' diagram overleaf)

> *Cambridge always recommend that you should consult your doctor before commencing any diet programme, but it is essential to get your doctor's signed confirmation of any medication or medical condition before you can start the 'Sole Source' programme, so that the doctor can adjust medication where appropriate.*

### *Step 1 – Sole Source*

The first programme is a nutritionally complete formula food (often referred to as a very low calorie diet, or the 'sole source of nutrition') which can be ideal for those who prefer a period of time away from the temptations of conventional food. Sole Source is suitable for those above BMI 25, with at least a stone (6.3kg) to lose.

On this programme, the dieter takes three Cambridge Diet meals in place of conventional food. For men, or women above 5ft 8ins (1.73m), four Cambridge Diet meals should be taken. In addition to water used to mix the diet powder and cups of unsweetened black tea or black coffee, it is advisable to drink at least 4pt (2.25ltr) of water per day.

Using the 'Sole Source' programme is not advisable when certain medical conditions are present. We say these conditions are 'contra-indicated'. There are also a number of medical conditions with which 'Sole Source' may be used with special precautions. These are detailed in Chapter 4 – The Vital Steps.

Cambridge recommends that the Sole Source programme is followed for no longer than four weeks at a time. At that point, if target weight has not yet been reached, the dieter should have an 'Add a Meal' week (see below)

# The 'Steps' Diagram

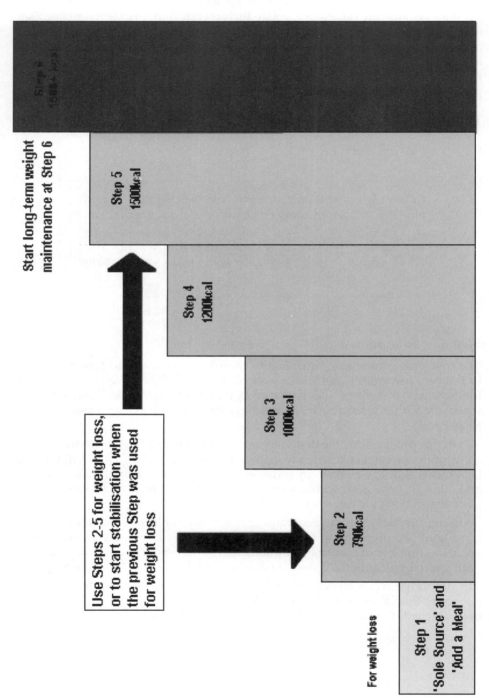

Start long-term weight maintenance at Step 6

Step 6
(1500+ kcal)

Step 5
1500kcal

Step 4
1200kcal

Step 3
1000kcal

Step 2
790kcal

Use Steps 2-5 for weight loss, or to start stabilisation when the previous Step was used for weight loss

For weight loss

Step 1
'Sole Source' and 'Add a Meal'

24

## Step 1 Add-a- Meal

The 'Add a Meal' menu is used as a natural break after four weeks on Sole Source, and is also the first part of the stabilisation process once target weight is achieved. Sometimes referred to as the 'green and white' meal, this menu introduces selected lean protein and vegetables to supplement the Cambridge meal options.

Three (or four) Cambridge options, plus a 3oz (80g) portion of white fish, poultry meat (without skin or fat), quorn or tofu, or skimmed milk cottage cheese. These can be accompanied by 2tbsp 'white or green' vegetables (cooked or raw) such as spring greens, cauliflower, lettuce, mushrooms, cabbage, courgettes or cucumber.

The dieter should continue to drink at least 4pt (2.25ltr)of water per day, and as much unsweetened black tea or black coffee as wished.

## Step 2 790 kcal

This weight loss programme combines nutritionally assured formula food with a healthy meal every day. It is ideal, for instance, for those who are unable to use 'Sole Source' for medical reasons. It is suitable for: those above BMI 25, or those below BMI 25 who may need a limited weight loss within a specific time scale (eg for a holiday or social event).

Similar to the 'Add-a-Meal' menu, except that only three Cambridge meals are taken, with the addition of a 6oz (150g) portion of poultry meat (without skin or fat), or an 8oz (250g) portion of white fish, quorn or tofu, or skimmed milk cottage cheese. These can be accompanied by 3tbsp 'white or green' vegetables (cooked or raw) such as spring greens, cauliflower, lettuce, mushrooms, cabbage, courgettes or cucumber. An additional allowance of ½ pint (235ml) skimmed milk is also allowed. The dieter should continue to drink at least 4pt (2.25ltr) of water per day, and as much unsweetened black tea or black coffee as wished.

## Step 3 1000 kcal

This programme adds fruit and carbohydrate to the 790 kcal meal described above. It is suitable for those who prefer to lose weight more gradually or those whose lifestyle makes it impossible to avoid conventional eating.

Two Cambridge meals plus 150 kcal breakfast of fruit, a portion of salad from 'white & green' vegetables listed above, the protein choices listed in Step 2 and an additional portion of carbohydrate. For example, 1½oz (40g) wholewheat pasta, noodles or rice, or 6oz (150g) boiled or baked potato. An extra 50 kcal allowance of fruit is allowed for dessert as well as of ½ pint (235ml) skimmed milk.

## Step 4 1200 kcal

This weight loss programme adds more selected conventional food to the daily menu. It is suitable for those who prefer to lose weight more gradually, or those whose lifestyle makes it impossible to avoid conventional eating.

Two Cambridge meal options, plus a 150 kcal portion of fruit for breakfast, a 300 kcal lunch and a 300 kcal main meal. Recommended menu choices for these meals are given in detail in Chapter 15.

## Step 5 1500 kcal

This weight loss programme adds more selected conventional food to the daily menu, whilst retaining a Cambridge meal for nutritional purposes. It is suitable for those who prefer to lose weight more gradually or those whose lifestyle makes it impossible to avoid conventional eating.

One Cambridge meal, 150 kcal fruit for breakfast; 350 kcal lunch and a 400 kcal main meal. Additional calorie allowances are made for snacks and desserts.

Although these are described as discrete steps, Cambridge can be used in a flexible way, and you can start on any step, using it as a preparation phase, before moving to a lower calorie level. The same calorie levels (steps) are also used after weight loss. It is here that the Cambridge programmes are most successful, because of the stabilisation and maintenance phases. When the target weight is reached, the dieter will continue to take Cambridge for nutrition and will gradually introduce selected conventional food over a period of several weeks. After this stabilisation period, the dieter will be at a healthy weight and can successfully maintain their new (lower) weight by choosing healthy portions of food through the guidance of their Counsellor.

The overall approach – where each Cambridge weight-loss programme comprises the four phases of preparation, weight-loss, stabilisation and maintenance – is explained in more detail in Chapter 3.

## Is it Safe?

It should be emphasised that Cambridge is not a 'fad' or 'crash' diet in any sense. Before it was marketed, eight years of research work went into its development and Cambridge has been used successfully by large numbers of people for long periods of time. Research on the diet started in 1970 at the West Middlesex Hospital, London, when Dr Ian McLean Baird and I decided to collaborate on the development of a new formula diet which could contain the fewest calories consistent with safety and good health.

Many of the popular diets recommended in magazines have very little scientific basis and very few have been tested in clinical trials. Both Dr Baird and I felt very strongly that before the Cambridge Diet was 'unleashed' on the general public, it should undergo the most rigorous testing, especially to establish its safety. We knew there would be scepticism and our professional reputations were at stake.

The diet was tested in much the same way as a new drug is. Many routine tests were conducted on hundreds of patients over long periods. No side effects of any major concern were encountered, and at the end of many years of study it was pronounced safe.

During the clinical trials, the Cambridge Diet was found to confer a number of distinct advantages. Among these were a decrease in blood fats and a lowering of blood pressure which in turn reduced the risk of coronary heart disease and stroke. The Diet was also found to be very suitable for overweight Type 2 diabetics, although it is important for a doctor to discontinue or adjust their usual medication.

Besides the extensive use of the Cambridge Diet for weight maintenance, many people – especially athletes – find it beneficial as a nutritional supplement, even where being overweight has never been a problem. Its regular consumption in the United States and Europe by hundreds of thousands of people for this purpose has established the Cambridge Diet as a staple foodstuff with many advantages. It is the most nutritionally dense food that exists, and contains all the basic nutrients required by man.

## For Better Health

In a civilization relying so much on manufactured and 'fast foods' (which are highly refined and often almost devoid of nutritional value), I believe such a complete foodstuff is needed to ensure adequate and balanced nutrition for those who are interested in obtaining it. Many expert nutritionists advocate eating a wide selection of different types of conventional food – what they call eating 'sensibly' – so as to include all the different nutrients in the correct amount we need. If people have the skill to plan their diet well, this can indeed be accomplished relatively easily and inexpensively. Few, however, devote the necessary time to such an important subject. How many people know how much zinc or copper they consumed yesterday, or today, or will consume tomorrow? To calculate the whole range of important nutrients in the foods you have eaten would take many hours – even using a computer.

From time to time, nutritional surveys are conducted into what various groups of people in the population – such as children, pregnant women, the elderly and minority ethnic groups – actually eat. The usual story is that there is some nutrient which is not being taken in adequate amounts. It may be vitamin C or A, or iron or copper. Very often it is found that different groups of people have different deficiencies, and that it is important for them to know what supplement or additional types of food they should be eating for perfect health. By consuming a complete foodstuff, like the Cambridge Diet, anyone can be sure that every nutrient is taken, in just the right amount, every day.

It is usual for people losing weight on a Cambridge programme to remark on how much better they feel. Of course, a lot of the benefit can be accounted for by their loss of weight. But it is equally due to the improvement in nutrition. Overweight people very often eat the wrong foods and are malnourished. Perhaps for the first time in their lives they are consuming the perfect food and understandably feel the benefit. Consequently they usually wish to continue with the diet as a nutritional supplement even after their ideal weight has been reached.

Cambridge programmes can make a major contribution towards the health of the nation, especially when combined with other behavioural changes. Government authorities now recommend that we eat fewer animal fats and less salt and sugar, and that we consume more fibre. By so doing, the incidence of. complaints such as coronary heart disease, stroke, diabetes and cancer can be greatly reduced. The Cambridge Counsellor makes a major contribution by drawing attention to these facts. The combination of a Cambridge weight management programme and sound nutritional principles can work together and help many people to live longer and healthier lives.

# The Whole Package

*3*

Commercial diets are often accused of failing. This is based on the premise that great numbers of people are on a diet at any one time, and that many people regain some of the weight they have lost. But no-one knows how many people are trying to lose weight, because a proper survey has never been carried out. One survey found that 32 percent of people they approached were trying to lose weight at the time. But 'trying' does not mean people were eating less; they may have just read a book on the subject; or thought they would start a diet – but not today!

The accusation that 'diets don't work' is unfair because most reputable, well-researched diets – if followed correctly – will help with weight loss. After that, people are on their own, and the fact that they regain weight is hardly the fault of the diet. This is where the Cambridge programmes differ, because everyone who tries one agrees to join a four-phase process:

☐ preparation
☐ weight loss
☐ stabilisation
☐ maintenance

Each of these is important for reasons explained below.

## Preparation

The significance of the Counsellor becomes immediately apparent right at the start. The first meeting between dieter and counsellor will establish a number of important factors about the person trying to lose weight because to have any chance of succeeding in the enterprise, both people will have to agree that the time is right. For example, the person's background – employment, family circumstances; their own weight history – will all have an impact on deciding whether now is a good time to begin such an undertaking. The dieter will need the support of friends and family.

Once this has been established, the preparation phase can be usefully used to reduce food intake gradually. This is particularly important for those on the 'Sole Source' programme, because the carbohydrate level is critical, and it is better to reduce the levels of carbohydrate, fats and sugar before the diet. A recommended approach is to begin on a programme that is one or two steps above that selected for weight loss, spending a few days (ideally a week) at each step. For example, if Step 2 (790 kcal) was going to be used for weight loss, the dieter could start on Step 4 (1200 kcal) for three days, then move down to Step3 (1000 kcal) for four days before starting the weight loss proper.

During this preparation phase, the dieter should gradually increase the amount of water they drink, and this is especially important for those who have a history of constipation. Those embarking on the Sole Source programme should also be made aware that whilst unlimited cups of coffee or tea may be taken, these drinks should be unsweetened and without milk. Those regular tea or coffee drinkers who cannot stand the thought of 'no milk' should start to reduce the amount of the beverage they drink, and take 'plain' water instead.

Using this kind of structured preparation is far better that the common scenario of starting a diet at 7am on a Monday morning – after one last massive fling over the weekend! This is just about the worse thing anyone could do, because decreasing carbohydrate intake so sharply could lead to withdrawal symptoms, including headaches and can increase tiredness and hunger. It is also very unhelpful because it will load glycogen stores and delay real weight loss.

Making a serious attempt to manage your weight is a big undertaking and represents a huge change in lifestyle. The preparation stage can also be used to try and pinpoint the underlying causes of the overweight problem: try and record typical daily intake; levels of activity; type of lifestyle – whether your job keeps you confined to a desk, or a car etc. The Counsellor will be able to help to identify those factors which can be changed, and will be able to offer the support and motivation to help the dieter decide that now is the time to change. Targeting smaller changes first can help a move towards being ready to lose weight.

Part of this decision will be based on the dieter's other commitments: there is little merit in planning to start immediately before a holiday period, for example. The amount of time spent in the weight loss stage will obviously depend on how much weight needs to be reduced, and which Cambridge programme will be used.

## Weight Loss

Surprisingly enough, the actual process of losing weight is probably the easiest part of the process.

Having chosen the day, look forward to it with pleasure. Tell yourself you are not going to feel hungry (if you do this you will not succumb to eating). If you live on your own, see that the house contains only the diet product and other specific foods you need for your Cambridge programme. If you live with a family, then keep the food out of sight and if you usually do the cooking, ask another member of the household to prepare the meals for the first day or two. It will be no problem once you are settled into your programme. Stick to the chosen Cambridge programme and the menu.

## Sole Source

On the Sole Source programme, this means that you will have thre
you are a man or above 5ft 8in) Cambridge meals – and *no oth*
*should also drink plenty of* water (I recommend at least eight glasses per day).

---

### Why So Much Water?

☐ Because food is largely composed of water (up to 70%), when you eat less, you also miss out on fluid. So, you need to drink extra water.

☐ Drinking more will help you to avoid potentially unpleasant side effects of dehydration, including muscle weakness, dizziness, headaches and bad moods.

☐ Drinking extra fluid will help your body to eliminate the waste products resulting from the breakdown of fat which happens as you lose weight.

☐ Drinking sufficient fluid will reduce the occurrence of constipation.

☐ Cambridge is a highly concentrated food, so drinking additional water will help to dilute the minerals to a more comfortable level of concentration.

---

Other allowable fluids include, black tea or coffee, tap or bottled water, which can be 'still' or 'sparkling', but should not contain fruit flavouring.

Forbidden fluids include: alcoholic beverages, milky tea or coffee, pure fruit juices and any drink containing sugar or calories.

The first three days on your diet will be very exciting, as you lose a great deal of weight every day. It is extremely exhilarating and highly motivating to continue. You will feel better and healthier than you have ever felt in your life because your body is receiving everything it needs.

Dependent on how you have prepared, you may feel hungry during the first three days, particularly during the evening. Either do something to keep your mind very occupied or go to bed early with a good book (or partner!). After a few days you will not feel hungry at all. Remember that if you do eat you will feel very hungry, because any extra food will stimulate your appetite. Make a commitment to lose weight and be determined!

### First Weeks

A few days after starting, you will suddenly realize that you are not hungry at all. In fact, you feel wonderful. Family and friends will comment on how happy you seem to be. You are in a state of euphoria! As long as you remain on the diet you will not be hungry and you will feel happy! If you are a housewife, then you will be able to prepare the family's food and serve them. If, while doing so, YOU experience a psychological desire for food, then have your Cambridge meal.

Because losing weight can be frustrating, especially during the first three days, the Cambridge Counsellor can be a great help to you and may make the difference between success and failure. If you have any problems or want advice, it is part of the Counsellor's job to help you.

You can indulge in all normal activities but you should not be unusually strenuous. Some people will feel a little tired; if you do, then sit down and take a rest.

You should weigh yourself every day at the same time, usually in the morning. You will be delighted with your progress and be very excited with it. This is the real motivation that makes you want to continue. As time goes on, and particularly at the end of the second week, you may experience several days when you do not lose weight. Do not become discouraged. It is very likely that you are losing fat but retaining water ; this is a process known as *plateauing*.

During this time you may be losing girth faster than weight. For this reason, we recommend that you use a tape measure to record your vital dimensions in addition to your weight. At this stage it is important for you to have faith in the diet because  – if you continue adhering to the diet – the weight-loss will restart once you lose the water you have been retaining.

As already mentioned, Cambridge is available in a number of different flavours and products. It is helpful to have different flavours throughout the day to avoid monotony.

## Stabilisation – The last few kilos

The Cambridge programmes from 790 to 1500 kcal are used for stabilisation as well as weight loss. In the stabilisation stage, your Cambridge meals are supplemented by the introduction of selected foods, which should not only help to ensure long-term weight maintenance, but will also prevent short-term weight regain. This stabilisation builds towards the final level of energy intake required to achieve a long-term stable weight.

Stabilisation should not be hurried. A **minimum** of a week should be spent on each Step – two weeks is better. The basic plan is to start stabilisation on the step above that which was used to lose weight. For example, if you used the Sole Source programme (Step 1) to lose weight, you should start stabilisation with 'Add a Meal', then move to Step 2 – 790 kcal and so on. The longer you spend at this phase, the more successful you will be in achieving a long-term stable – and maintainable – weight.

If the recommendations are followed to the letter then you should continue to shed a little more weight during this period of stabilisation. For this reason, there is no need to go below target weight to allow for rebound weight-gain as there will be none once weight loss has stopped.

## Weight Maintenance

Maintenance usually begins when there is neither weight gain nor weight loss, and can start at about 1500 kcal per day. However, it will vary from person to person: because the recommended daily energy intake figures are 2000 kcal for women and 2500 kcal for men, some people may still lose some weight if their intake is below these levels.

The problem is that there is a danger that – after the 'exciting' weight loss phase has been achieved – all the old reasons for being overweight could return.

This won't be the case if you followed the stabilisation programme and come to understand the reasons for your original overweight. Maintenance consists of taking practical steps to maintain your new weight by selecting healthy food choices and by increasing the levels of activity. Many people continue to use Cambridge once or twice a day – not only to control energy intake but to carry on getting the benefits of good nutrition.

Keep a regular check on your weight. When your body weight is increased by more than five pounds above your ideal weight, it is time to take prompt action. This can be done by cutting out a conventional meal and having a Cambridge meal instead. As time goes by, people who have been plagued by being overweight for most of their lives become slim, and attain great confidence. The Cambridge Diet is a very powerful tool with which you can control your weight.

## Cutting Down on the Calories

You became overweight because you consumed more calories than your body needed. So, to maintain your new weight, you must change your eating habits for ever. If you return to your habit of eating, say, 3000 kcal per day, then you will soon regain the weight you have lost.

You may be one of those extremely clever people who, armed with a calculator, can immediately tot up the calorie content of each meal. If you are like me, you plan your meals according to broad principles and tackle the problem by avoiding foods of high calorie value. In this respect, you will find the following hints helpful.

---

**Tips for Weight Maintenance**

avoid fat
restrict salt
restrict sugar
restrict alcohol
eat fibre

---

### Avoid fat

☐ Fat (and oils) contain nine calories per gram, which is two and a quarter times more than protein or carbohydrate. If you are to control your weight, it is extremely important that you restrict the quantities of fat and oils that you eat.

☐ Avoid fried foods and fatty foods. Wherever possible, grill and poach but rarely fry. (If you do need to fry, use a nonstick pan.) Especially avoid fried chips (French fries), potato crisps and food fried in batter. Eat boiled and poached, rather than fried eggs.

☐ When vegetables are cooked, do not mix them with butter.

☐ With salads, use a low-calorie salad dressing, vinegar or lemon juice, herbs and spices.

☐ Avoid foods made with pastry such as meat and fruit pies, fatty croissants, Danish pastries, and sausage rolls.

☐ Use skimmed milk instead of full cream milk. Use low fat yoghurt instead of cream.

☐ Use low fat cheese (e.g. cottage cheese) and have cream and hard cheese just occasionally.

☐ Use less butter and margarine on bread.

☐ Eat nuts occasionally but never more than a two-ounce packet at a time (they are very high in calories).

☐ Use lean cuts of meat and wherever possible cut the fat off meat and eat only the lean part.

☐ Eat grilled chicken, without the skin, and white fish more frequently, since these are less fatty.

## Restrict salt

Too much salt in the diet can cause high blood pressure and fluid retention.

☐ Avoid, as far as possible, adding salt at the table. If you have to use any at all, substitute one of the new mineral salts (in which part of the salt is replaced by potassium salts).

☐ Most of the salt we eat is put into manufactured (e.g. canned and packaged) foods. Thus use unsalted, rather than salted butter, and also unsalted nuts. Eat little salty fish (kippers, smoked and canned fish) and potato crisps. When cooking your own cakes and pastries or Yorkshire pudding go easy on the salt and use the special mineral salt referred to above.

## Eat fibre

Fruit and vegetables and wholemeal bread contain a lot of roughage (fibre). Special crispbreads and crisps containing bran are also recommended. Besides filling you up and curbing your appetite, they're healthy.

## Restrict sugar

Although sugar is not as calorific as fat or alcohol, it is still a highly concentrated source of calories, with no other nutritional value. Avoid sugar drinks (cordials, sweet fizzy sodas and Cola). Use one of the low-calorie varieties instead. If you must sweeten coffee or tea use a sugar substitute with one of the calorie-free sweeteners, such as saccharine or aspartame, which is indistinguishable from sugar and leaves no aftertaste. Most of the sweeteners are unstable if heated, so if you are sweetening stewed fruit, the sweetener should be added after cooking and not before.

In many manufactured foods, sugar is often combined with fat. Sweets, chocolate and creamy cakes should be treated with suspicion!

## Alcohol

Drink only in moderation, since alcohol contains seven calories per gram (one and three-quarter times more than carbohydrate or protein). Health authorities in the UK recommend limiting the consumption of alcohol to 21 units per week for men and 14 units for women. A unit is defined as one 125ml glass of wine, 300ml beer, or one 25ml measure of spirits.

There is now a large body of evidence that moderate alcohol drinking especially of red wine is beneficial and increases life span. However, excessive alcohol – besides piling on the calories – is very deleterious and has the opposite effect. The standard advice if you are a drinker is to restrict your consumption to the sensible amounts given above.

☐ Limit your drinking to no more than one or two drinks per day. If you drink at lunch time, skip it for dinner.

☐ Mineral water with ice and a slice of lemon makes an excellent drink at parties and is even fashionable nowadays.

## Eating out

In his book 'Fat Land', Greg Critser explains how Americans became the fattest people in the world. During the last 40 years, the consumption of fast food (hamburgers, fried chicken, french fries, Tex Mex food etc ) in USA has increased enormously. In order to promote their sales and to compete with others, the portion sizes have increased dramatically over the years. For instance, what was a typical fast food meal of 610 kcal  in 1960 exploded to 1550 calories in 2003. Since so many Americans eat out, it is not surprising why they have become fatter. In Europe , the British are now the most overweight and obese and there is no doubt that the increase in the consumption of 'Fast Food' and the portion sizes has contributed.

My advice is to avoid 'Fast Food' if at all possible. If you have to eat out regularly, choose those outlets where you can limit your calories by carefully selecting suitable food which fits in with the good nutritional  principles given above. If I had to make a choice I would buy a sandwich and have a glass of semi-skimmed milk or tea or coffee.But take care to look at the calorie count on the packet because some sandwiches are loaded with mayonnaise and can have twice as many calories as others.

## Healthy Eating

At this point you will have reached the conclusion that everything you like is strictly taboo and fattening. You may be one of those people who loves fish and chips, cream gateaux and salty hamburgers with French fries. How is it possible to eat sensibly and lead a happy life? There is a sensible approach, which I adopt myself.

Most of the time, about six days a week, I am fairly strict and eat very sensibly, according to the above rules. Then once a week I will throw caution to the winds and indulge. Now and again I will have fish and chips and enjoy it tremendously. The same applies to sccnes with strawberry jam and cream. Most nutritionists I know do exactly the same. Treats are even more enjoyable if they're not everyday events!

## Recommended Menus

To help you in your search for interesting and tasty food, Chapter 15 provides a number of practical low-calorie menus. These are designed to complement Cambridge during the stabilisation and maintenance phases, and they are also a helpful guide to the type of dishes you should be eating as part of your permanent eating plan.

## The Secret

The secret of keeping weight off is that Cambridge is always available whenever you need it. In our original experiments at the West Middlesex Hospital, one lady originally weighing 22st 12lb (320lb - 145kg) lost about 11st (154lb - 70kg) in hospital. While there, she was adamant that she would never regain her weight, having spent one year of her life in hospital losing it. But she didn't.

Unfortunately, after discharge she moved to another part of the country and it became impossible to contact her. Two years later, she turned up at the hospital having regained all the weight she had lost, and was even heavier.

There were no supplies of Cambridge Diet available for her maintenance programme in those days. If we were dealing with her case today, I believe it would be a different story, as shown by countless others who have followed her, but have succeeded in keeping slim.

Also, of course, if someone weighs, say 15st (210lb - 95kg) then reduces to 12st (168lb - 76kg) but gradually increases back to perhaps 14st (196lb - 89kg) over a period of years, there has still been a health benefit; without the earlier weight loss, the person may have increased to 19st (266lb - 120kg) and been subject to greatly increased health hazards.

## A Permanent Change

One of the most severe criticisms of the Cambridge Diet made by some psychologists and hospital dieticians, is that it does not change people's eating habits in the long term and is therefore useless, particularly for maintaining weight-loss. To these armchair critics it is just another fad diet. Nothing could be further from the truth as anyone can vouch who has used the diet as a sole source of nutrition for several weeks. For the first time one realizes that vast quantities of food are not indispensable to life. It trains you to live without having food continually on your mind and the experience has a beneficial effect on most people. There is ample proof that the Cambridge stabilisation maintenance plan achieves excellent results in returning the dieter to long-term healthy eating principles.

# The Vital Steps

## Seeing Your Doctor

Anyone thinking of weight loss should see their doctor before starting **any** diet.

In the case of Cambridge, tell him or her that you intend to use one of the Cambridge weight management programmes. Your Cambridge Counsellor will be able to supply you with an "Information for Doctors" booklet and other literature which explains each programme if any queries are raised.

If you are on medication, or have a medical condition, your doctor will be asked to confirm what this is as it may affect which programmes are best for you, or whether the medication needs to be monitored or adjusted.

Despite its success around the world, Cambridge is not suitable for everyone and one of the first things that you will discuss with your Counsellor is whether or not there is a Cambridge programme that you can use. Cambridge have devised the following four safety categories:

| Medication Safety Categories | |
| --- | --- |
| A  contraindicated | you should not use any programme |
| B  not low calorie | you should only use programmes above 1000kcal |
| C  special precaution | you can use any programme, although your doctor may need to adjust medication |
| D  other medication | you can use any programme |

## A – Contraindicated

There are certain people who should not use any Cambridge (or indeed any other!)weight loss programme – unless under medical supervision. They include *pregnant women* and those who are *breast feeding* or have *given birth within the previous 3 months*. Also excluded *are children below the age of fourteen*. The reason for these exclusions is that the protein requirements of people in these categories are much higher than normal, and the diet would not supply them with enough of this vital nutrient. However, if your doctor decides that despite these circumstances you should lose weight, then it is possible to use

Cambridge as part of a supervised diet which contains more calories than the Cambridge Diet does on its own.

Other people who need higher than normal levels of protein are those who have had a heart attack or stroke within the previous 3 months, or who are recovering from an operation or serious accident which occurred during the same period.

There are a number of serious or severe chronic conditions which would also rule against you using a Cambridge weight loss programme, and these include serious heart conditions; severe liver or kidney disease and severe depression.

Also to be considered are the *elderly*. Many overweight people in their seventies have lost a great deal of weight on the Cambridge Diet, and age by itself does not debar people from using it. The doctor should advise, and caution may be required if person suffers from postural hypotension.

## Contraindications

☐ pregnant or breast feeding women

☐ children below 14

☐ anyone who (within previous 3 months) has had
- ◆ heart attack
- ◆ stroke
- ◆ serious accident
- ◆ operation

☐ anyone who suffers with
- ◆ serious heart condition
- ◆ severe kidney disease
- ◆ severe liver disease
- ◆ severe depression
- ◆ porphyria
- ◆ anorexia nervosa or bulimia nervosa

☐ anyone taking the following medication:
- ◆ insulin
- ◆ anti-obesity drugs

Type 1 diabetics who are taking insulin are contraindicated because of the problems of regulating blood sugar levels. Fortunately, very few Type 1 sufferers are overweight. The other type of medication that is contraindicated are the anti-obesity drugs and their use should not be continued.

## B – Not Low Calorie

The blood levels of people taking medications in this category are very important to successful treatment, and therefore we restrict the use of Cambridge programmes to those above 1000kcal per day. This category includes four sub-groups:

☐ anti-coagulants

☐ anti-arrhythmia

☐ anti-convulsants

☐ lithium

### Anti-coagulants

Anti-coagulants, anti-thrombotics and fibrolytics all reduce the clotting time of blood. They are frequently prescribed following open heart surgery, heart attacks, deep vein thrombosis or arterial thrombosis. The blood levels of these medicines are of critical importance to successful treatment. A reduced calorie intake will allow them to be more quickly absorbed into the bloodstream and could upset this delicate balance.

### Anti-arrhythmia (Digoxin)

This medicine is used to correct irregularities in the heart rate associated with heart failure. The blood levels of this medicine are normally difficult to balance. A reduced calorie intake could increase this instability by allowing more rapid absorption.

### Anti-convulsants

Anti-convulsant drugs are used to treat epilepsy and seizures. Epilepsy results from an altered neurochemical state that leads to excess electrical activity in the brain. The fluid and electrolyte changes brought about by the natural diuretic effect of the Cambridge Diet may alter dosage requirements. Treatments are aimed at controlling this activity. There is always a gradual increase or decrease in medication according to need, and it is finely tuned. A reduced calorie intake will increase the absorption rate of this medicine into the blood stream and may interfere with the desired treatment levels.

### Lithium

Lithium is used to treat severe psychiatric disorders. A reduced calorie intake will increase the absorption rate of this drug which may alter the blood levels. As a constant level is essential for successful treatment and to prevent toxic effects occurring, it should not be used with the Cambridge Diet.

## C – Special Precautions

Because of the low calorific level in the Cambridge Diet, people taking certain medicines may need their doctor to adjust the dosage level and, in some cases, the doctor may need to discontinue medication completely. Customers in this group should have their progress monitored by their doctor. These medications are:

☐ anti-hypertensives

☐ diuretics

☐ oral hypoglycaemics

☐ gout prevention

### Anti-hypertensives

Anti-hypertensive drugs are used to reduce all grades of raised blood pressure. This group includes beta-blockers, ace inhibitors, calcium antagonists, vasodilators, alpha-blockers, central alpha agonists and diuretics. Some medicines appear in both this and the next section (diuretics) because they are combinations of two different medicines – for example, a beta-blocker with a diuretic or two different diuretics.

For those on a programme below 1200kcal per day, it is advisable to discontinue diuretics, whilst the dosage of the other drugs in this group needs to be reduced before starting Cambridge. For some customers, regular blood pressure checks and blood tests (such as kidney function tests and serum potassium levels) may be advisable. The doctor may then need to adjust the dosage accordingly.

The reason for this recommendation is that the reduced calorie intake will bring about a reduction in blood pressure. Provided that fluid levels are kept high, there should not be a problem. However, the low calorie weight loss programme together with hypertensive medication may make the blood pressure drop too low if the dosage is not adjusted.

### Diuretics

Diuretics (water tablets) are frequently used for the treatment of mild to moderate high blood pressure (hypertension). It is advisable for the doctor to stop a customer's diuretic medication before the Cambridge Diet is begun. A reduced calorie intake brings about a natural water-loss effect, which can also occur with diuretics. The effect of the two together would not only cause too much water to be lost with the risk of dehydration, but more importantly – the loss of an important body salt, potassium. Potassium – an electrolyte – stimulates muscle action, and too much loss could affect the heart. When prescribing diuretics doctors usually monitor a patients potassium levels or prescribe potassium sparing medication.

## Oral hypoglycaemics

These are given to treat Type II (mature onset) diabetes. Customers on anti-diabetic tablets should ideally have their medication discontinued by their doctor while on 'Sole Source'. Regular blood sugar checks should be performed in the first few days of dieting and thereafter at weekly intervals. Sole Source lowers blood sugar levels and the combination with hypoglycaemic medication could make the blood sugar levels drop too low.

## Gout prevention

All VLCDs produce a rise in serum uric acid levels during the first two weeks, which may lead to an acute attack of gout in known sufferers. Preventative treatment with an uricosuric agent should be given concurrently with the Cambridge Diet from the day of commencement.

## D – Other Medications

People taking other medications may use any Cambridge weight loss programme.

## Side Effects on 'Sole Source'

It is unusual for people to experience side effects from using the Cambridge Sole Source programme, but a few do have some minor problems, especially during the first three days. Most of these problems are common to all diets and have short-term remedies as listed below:

## Headaches

Headaches may occur due to dehydration or, more rarely, because of carbohydrate or caffeine withdrawal. An increase in fluid intake should help, but take a pain-killer if necessary.

## Constipation

Since the diet contains only a small amount of bulk you will find that bowel movements are less frequent. However, if you are suffering discomfort due to constipation, then a natural laxative, such as Fybogel (available from chemists) may be taken according to instructions. In the UK and some other countries, Cambridge drinks and soups contain inulin – a natural vegetable fibre – which reduces the likelihood of constipation. Cambridge Fibre'89 can also be added to any food or drink and is undetectable in taste or texture.

## Nausea and diarrhoea

These symptoms may occur as a result of not drinking enough water. In addition to the liquid in which your diet is made up, you should also drink at least 4pt (2.25ltr) of water a day. The Cambridge Diet contains concentrated minerals and vitamins which may make you feel sick if they are not diluted with water. Drink plenty of liquid after consuming the Cambridge Diet. For instance, you should always have a glass of water or a cup of black tea or coffee or low calorie drink immediately afterwards. Alternatively, you could take the Diet in six (or eight) half portions at regular intervals. If the symptoms do not settle down, the Diet should be discontinued, or a programme 'with food' selected.

## Dizziness

Dizziness is most often caused by the diuretic effect of the diet. Drink plenty of water and you will find that it will usually disappear. For those who are prone to attacks of faintness, it is important to avoid what is called postural hypertension'. This occurs when one rises from a chair too rapidly and feels faint and dizzy. In such circumstances, remember not to rush up quickly from your sitting position but to take life a little more slowly!

## Mouth odour

After you have been on the diet sole source for a few days your family and friends may tell you that your breath smells. The reason why it happens is that since you have stopped eating your mouth is not being completely cleaned by the food you chew. A partial solution is to brush your teeth often and to use a mouthwash frequently. There is also available low calorie chewing gum (not ordinary gum) which will achieve the cleansing effect of food.

## Fatigue

Some people who lead a very strenuous life and are used to a job which is physically demanding, or alternatively play vigorous games, find that they are more fatigued than usual for a short time. The solution here is to take life a bit easier and perhaps go to bed earlier. On the other hand, many people who are not used to a strenuous life find that they have a good deal more energy and can achieve much more physically than they did before going on the diet.

## Irritability

Most people feel very happy whilst taking the Cambridge Diet, but occasionally there are those who feel slightly irritable. This is usually at the beginning of the diet and with time the effect wears off and one's mood changes for the better.

## Other Side Effects

Over the last 20 years there have been a handful of reports of other side effects, which include:

### Hair Loss

Hair loss, with a generalised thinning of the hair, is usually linked to emotional stress, severe illness, malnutrition, hypothyroidism, hormones, and (for a few people) extensive weight loss over a sustained period of time whatever the method of weight loss used. So, it is due to a physiological response to the actual weight loss process rather than to the Diet. You can be reassured that the incidence of hair loss is very low, and that hair does re-grow, usually thicker and glossier than before. It is the "lesser of the evils" and you will have the best of both worlds – a healthy weight and a good head of hair.

*This condition should not be confused with alopecia whereby hair comes out in patches which is a medical condition needing treatment by a doctor.*

### Impaired vision

Very rarely, a temporary change in vision shows up if a routine eye test is performed during the weight loss phase. It can happen if the customer is not drinking enough while using the 'Sole Source' programme. In such cases, the lack of fluid in the body causes a loss of fluid from inside the eye, thereby slightly affecting its shape. The remedy is to drink more water, which should restore the correct shape to the eyeball. The effect is self-righting once 'Sole Source' is finished and does not present a long-term problem.

### Cramp

A few people are prone to cramp while using the 'Sole Source' programme. It is not caused by the diet itself, but by the increased throughput of fluid in the body's tissues. The muscle spasms result from changes in sodium levels as the water shifts between cells. Keep warm and try a drink of slimline tonic water just before bedtime. The quinine content may offer relief – as may "Crampex" tablets.

### Reduced body temperature

Feeling chilly is almost certainly due to the reduced food intake. When someone eats a large, conventional meal, the body generates a lot of body heat; clearly, as the intake energy level drops, so too does the amount of body heat generated. Individuals can differ widely in this – known as 'thermogenic response'.

For those that are affected, the cold feeling is due to the very small number of calories on the Sole Source programme. Other factors that influence body heat production include the slight reduction in metabolic rate which always happens during weight loss, and of course the loss of insulating fat! If you are sensitive to the cold, you should try to move around more and wrap up warmly: a number of light layers are more effective than a single heavy layer.

43

## Rashes

Skin Rashes can be caused by any number of things – pollution, temperature, sunlight, fabrics, washing powders, etc – as well as food. However, just occasionally, there is something in the formula of the Cambridge Diet to which someone has an allergic reaction. Stop, then restart the programme to ascertain whether Cambridge is the cause, and contact your Counsellor who may be able to help. If Cambridge is thought to be the cause, it may not be suitable for you, although you could try an alternative product (eg a Tetra Brik, or avoid the meal bars etc).

## Menstrual cycle

Whenever someone's body changes in weight it will be accompanied by fluctuation in the hormone levels – particularly in women. For most women, the menstrual cycle is not affected, but some will experience increased activity and break-through bleeding, whilst others may find that their periods stop for a while. Any hormone fluctuations will stop once target weight is reached. When the body ceases to lose weight, the metabolic rate will settle – to a new level appropriate to the new weight – and consequently the hormones will also settle down and find their own pattern again.

## Skinfolds

Whenever someone successfully loses a large amount of weight – on any weight loss programme – they may find that their skin may sag. It should recover, but the speed of recovery will depend on the dieter's age, general health and level of nutrition. Ageing reduces the amount of collagen – the main support structure in the skin – making it less supple with time. Younger skin will therefore firm up more quickly than older skin following weight loss. It is unusual for there to be no reduction in skinfolds once weight has stabilised for a prolonged period of time. Although nothing can regenerate lost collagen, massaging with lotions and oils may help, whilst a well-balanced diet will encourage good health in general and will contribute to a healthy, glowing skin. The complete, balanced and easily absorbed nutrition in the Cambridge Diet seems to speed up the process of firming skin and reduce skinfolds. Increasing activity levels and specific exercises to tone the body will also help.

## Persistent side effects

The advantage of losing weight should certainly override any short-term discomfort you may experience. However, should the side effects continue it is important to consult your Cambridge Counsellor or doctor for further advice.

# The Cambridge Counsellor 5

## Friendly Support

Anyone who has tried dieting will know that the hardest part is not starting but keeping going. Motivation is such a key component to success, which is why so many of the people who give up before hitting their target weight tell of how little help they got from friends and family.

Why is this? Why do partners – who are quick to grumble about their opposite number being fatter than they should be – do so little to help reverse the situation? Perhaps it is because of disruption to normal family life; or because they have to give up their favourite foods. Perhaps they resent the centre of attention being focused on someone else. Whatever the reason, this lack of support can put paid to good intentions.

With experience of the Cambridge Diet from all round the world, there's no doubt that the best results are achieved when the programme is directed by someone trained to understand the problems associated with losing weight and who has ample time – more time than just 5 or 10 minutes – in which to provide adequate levels of support.

## The Counsellor Edge

This is where a Cambridge Counsellor provides an edge over other dietary methods. Through the Counsellor's help, the dieter gets all the personal support and one-to-one advice they need.

In the UK, Cambridge programmes and products are only available through a Cambridge Counsellor, many of whom liaise closely with their local health professionals. Each is an independent, self-employed business, acting as their own, small-scale slimming centre. Although Cambridge Counsellors are all different, they have two things in common. The first is that **all of them** have used the Diet for at least a couple of weeks. And the second is that the **vast majority** of them have successfully lost weight through the use of the Diet.

So, the Counsellor – the person you are relying on for advice and guidance – is doing so from first-hand experience and not from a theoretical textbook. Who else would be better placed to help others? Those who have succeeded the Cambridge way are usually only too delighted to help others. And enthusiasm is contagious!

## Sponsorship

For this reason, most new Counsellors join the Cambridge organisation through the recommendation of an existing Counsellor. However, before they are accepted and accredited, there is an extensive Company training programme they must go through to ensure they have the necessary knowledge they need to back up their personal experience.

They must also demonstrate that they are committed to providing a high level of service to their clients. The process of slimming can be a very emotional period with the occasional depressions along with the high spots. The most successful Counsellors are those who are always there for their clients – even if this is officially "out of hours".

Not surprisingly, the role of Counsellor tends to attract those who enjoy communicating. They may come from any walk of life, but the most important quality is a genuine interest in people and a desire to help others. The most successful are not necessarily those with the most qualifications but the ones with the biggest hearts.

## Training for Counsellors

Counsellors shouldn't be mistaken for doctors, nurses or nutritionists, and it is unreasonable and unfair to expect them to comment on these kinds of matters. Instead, they are trained to have a high level of knowledge about the programmes and how they can best be used. They receive their training from the Company and other senior Counsellors, through seminars and conferences and through Company literature and books. All new Counsellors have successfully to complete a product knowledge test and a telephone accreditation interview.

Further training is undertaken by attendance at training conferences and through the Cambridge Counsellor Development scheme, which comprise a number of separate modules. These modules, which are designed to be completed by the Counsellor at home, cover a range of relevant topics, from counselling skills, basic nutrition and health, medical matters and latest information on Cambridge programmes and products.

## Links with Health Professionals

Although we said earlier that Counsellors are not health professionals, we should say that some health professionals are Cambridge Counsellors. In addition to these, Cambridge operates a programme specifically designed for the Primary or Secondary Care environment, in which specially trained and accredited Counsellors work alongside health professionals in the management of their obese and medically compromised patients. These Counsellors are known as Cambridge Primary Care Counsellors (PCCs).

Health professionals regard the PCCs and the clinically proven Cambridge programmes as a viable option, providing them – and their patients – with a valuable intervention in the treatment of obesity. They are a welcome addition to many over stretched and under resourced practices.

Delivery and implementation of the weight care programmes are flexible. Patients can attend a weekly Cambridge Weight Care Clinic at the practice, or visit the PCC at their home. Each practice can select their preferred method to suit a patient's particular requirements and circumstances.

## Code of Conduct

As part of our commitment towards customer care, all UK Counsellors agree to follow a Code of Conduct, which provides clear guidelines, and also ensures that their customers know what to expect from them throughout their weight management programme. It outlines the minimum acceptable standards of Counselling which will ensure correct, responsible and safe practices.

The Code of Conduct covers a range of topics, including contact with dieters, the importance of the screening interview, and the continuing role of the Counsellor throughout the four phases of any weight loss programme.

## The Support Role

Every Counsellor has personal experience of using the Cambridge Diet, and wants to use their knowledge and skills to help others manage their own weight. After a period of training with their sponsor, they are accredited by the Company Medical Officer and are then ready to begin their own independent business whose aim is

☐ to provide advice and support during all stages of the Weight Care programme

☐ to supply a full range of products

☐ to advise and help motivate customers towards a healthier lifestyle based on sound, balanced nutrition

In order to provide a personal, safe service, the Counsellor conducts a screening interview to determine the dieter's weight and measurements and whether they have a medical condition or are taking medication. In these cases, the customer's doctor is asked to verify the information. These details are noted on a Medical Record Form, which is signed by the customer. In every case, Cambridge recommend that the customer's doctor is notified when starting a weight loss programme, and is kept informed about progress.

## Around the World

Elsewhere around the world, Cambridge is distributed in a variety of ways appropriate to local requirements, but all retain the support element which has been a fundamental part of the success story.

This could be provided by a trained dietician in a clinic setting; by personalised advice and treatments in fitness and beautician salons; or through trained staff in a pharmacy or health food store, backed by information and literature designed for both staff and customers.

# The Nutritional Benefits

6

There is more to a healthy life than just being thin. Many of the diseases which affect our lives are due to faulty nutrition. Among them are coronary heart disease, high blood pressure, stroke and cancer. All these diseases occur in thin as well as fat people. Also, nutritional surveys have shown that many people do not consume the recommended level of many vitamins, minerals and trace elements. It is common for obese people to comment that after weight reduction they feel fitter and healthier than they have ever done in their life. They continue to take Cambridge meals, not only for weight maintenance, but as a nutritional supplement, as it contains all the recommended daily allowances of the above nutrients.

Even naturally thin people take Cambridge just for nutrition. By doing so, they are using good nutrition to help to prevent diseases occurring.

There are a number of very good reasons why the Cambridge Diet is potentially beneficial in prolonging life and it fits in well with modern concepts of the perfect nutritional lifestyle.

## Coronary Heart Disease

There is still much controversy on this subject in the scientific and medical world and it is not surprising that the public is often very confused. Briefly, animal fats including dairy products and meat fats, etc., raise the level of a substance in the blood called cholesterol. It is this substance which accumulates in the inner walls of arteries, notably in the coronary arteries. Those people who are susceptible to attacks of coronary thrombosis often, but not always, have a high level of blood cholesterol. Vegetable oils, like corn, sunflower seed and safflower oil are thought to lower the level of blood cholesterol. For this reason, many nutritionists recommend that these replace animal fats. Vegetable oils are rich in what are called polyunsaturated fatty acids and the animal fats are rich in saturated fats.

In industrialized countries, the total consumption of fat is about 40 per cent of all the calories eaten. Public health authorities recommend that it should be reduced to about 30 per cent, and some authorities suggest even lower levels. The PS ratio of the fat consumed should be increased. That means that the proportion of polyunsaturated (present in vegetable oils) to saturated fatty acids (present in animal fats) should be increased.

The Cambridge Diet contains no animal fats aside from the small amounts in skimmed milk.. In fact, it is very low in fat and contains only 3 grams per day, of which two-thirds is polyunsaturated. If one were recommending a diet which would be suitable as a prevention for coronary heart disease, the Cambridge Diet would take top place. It contributes virtually no fats to the total intake and when eaten with other low fat foods would be instrumental in cutting down the total fat calories to those which are recommended.

Cambridge is also cholesterol free. And, although many people believe that dietary cholesterol is not important, some nutritionists recommend that food rich in cholesterol should be avoided.

## High Blood Pressure

The incidence of high blood pressure in the population is increasing, partly because people are living longer and blood pressure increases with age. High blood pressure causes damage in two ways; either by precipitating coronary heart disease or by causing stroke. Thus a control of your blood pressure is extremely important if these two diseases are to be prevented. Most experts agree that the main nutritional factors which could contribute to high blood pressure are:

☐   too much salt in the diet

☐   not enough potassium

☐   too little polyunsaturated fats

☐   excessive alcohol intake

Much of our knowledge of these factors comes from population studies. For instance, some Japanese eat vast quantities of salt daily, because it is used in the preservation of the fish they eat. They can consume as much as 20 to 35 grams of salt per day. Their most prevalent cause of death is stroke, caused by very high blood pressure.

It has been suggested that the epidemic of high blood pressure in industrialized countries could be prevented if the salt content could be reduced drastically. Health authorities recommend that the current intake of about 12 grams per day should be reduced to one-third, about four grams per day. It is interesting that potassium salts counteract this effect of salt and there is a move towards increasing its intake.

The Cambridge Diet makes an important contribution in this area. It contains only 1.4 grams of sodium per day but is very high in potassium (2.5 grams per day). This means that it is a moderately low sodium, high potassium diet. Although it does contain some polyunsaturated fatty acids, which are also beneficial towards lowering blood pressure, these are in rather small amounts. Therefore, it is important to supplement the Cambridge Diet with vegetable oils – for example corn oil – when on the maintenance programme.

It is only a high intake of alcohol which increases blood pressure, and one or two drinks a day have no effect whatever. Thus, if you think it is important to drink alcohol – and some research suggests that a moderate daily consumption of red wine is beneficial – you should not exceed this quantity, otherwise you may risk increasing your blood pressure.

# Cancer

Our knowledge of the importance of nutrition in the prevention of cancer has increased remarkably during the last few years. The nutrients which appear to be involved are; dietary fat, fibre, vitamins A, C and E, and also selenium. A high level of fat in the diet seems to be related to a higher incidence of cancer in animals. In this respect, vegetable oils are no different and may be even worse than animal fats. For this reason, many health authorities recommend that the total fat consumption should be reduced and there should be no net increase in vegetable oils. Therefore, a decrease in total fat levels could be of great value in the prevention of two major diseases which affect us; coronary heart disease and cancer.

In experimental studies in animals, it is found that vitamin E and selenium can stop the formation of chemical substances known as 'free radicals', because they are antioxidants (prevent oxidation). There is one important theory which states that free radicals are one of the major promoters of cancer in the body and any measure which cuts down their formation is worthwhile. The Cambridge Diet provides ample vitamin E and selenium. Also, in animals, vitamin A has been found to be very effective in preventing cancers caused by the introduction of cancer-forming substances. The vitamin apparently works by affecting the surfaces of cells so that they are less susceptible to other substances which may cause cancer.

Vitamin C works in a different way. Many foodstuffs contain nitrites as preservatives. When nitrites enter the stomach they are converted into cancer-forming substances called nitrosamines. Vitamin C prevents the formation of these nitrosamines and has been shown to be very effective experimentally in animals.

To summarize, the high vitamin A, C, E and selenium content of the Cambridge Diet is potentially very useful if it is indeed the case that vitamins and minerals can help to prevent cancer.

Dietary fibre is also thought by some experts to prevent colon cancer. For this reason maybe it is important to include fibre in a maintenance diet, as suggested above.

# Longevity

Although many people are now living to a greater age, the natural life span, that is the maximum time people live, is still no more than it was 100 years ago. Most people die in their seventies or eighties, and although more people now reach that age, the total life span is not increasing.

During the last century, people died young from the infectious diseases, such as tuberculosis, pneumonia and cholera, which were rife within the population because of poor public health standards. With the greater awareness of the causes of these diseases and the introduction of antibiotics, very few people now die from them. However, as more people live longer, they die from diseases of old age, or more particularly from coronary heart disease, cancer and stroke.

A major question for the future is whether it will be possible to increase the life span to 100 or 120 years or even more. One physician, Dr J. Walford of UCLA, believes it may he possible to do this. He expresses his view in a book, *Maximum Life Span*. The method he suggests is to eat less – much less. His theory is based on work on experimental animals. For instance, rats which are fed on about 50 per cent of what they normally eat, increase their life span up to 60 per cent, providing that the diet still contains adequate vitamins, minerals and other important nutrients. In other words, the secret of longevity is 'under-nutrition' without malnutrition. Other scientists have shown that intermittent fasting (that is, cutting out food for a few days) also has an effect on increasing life span in rats. Animals fed a high quality diet, as much as they wanted, but made to fast completely every second day, lived over 1,000 days compared with only 800 days for those which had normal rations.

How can a decreased intake of foods increase your life span? The answer may lie in your body temperature. Animals kept in a cool temperature live much longer than those who are warm. This happens when you go without food. Your body temperature decreases and your metabolism is slowed down. These are the two factors which are thought to increase life span.

Dr Walford recommends a total abstinence from food for two successive days every week and a healthy moderate diet during the other five days. When not eating food, it is important to take other non-calorific nutrients, such as vitamins, minerals and trace elements. If one were looking for a diet which would fit in with his concept, it would be the Cambridge Sole Source programme. There are many people who are taking it not only twice a week sole source, but very often five days or more. If Dr Walford is right, then people who carry out this regime over many years should live a great deal longer. Time will tell if he is right!

## Cambridge as a Nutritional Supplement

There are many of us who believe that the most important contribution that Cambridge can make to all our lives is to provide good, basic nutrition. Three Cambridge meals every day will provide all the recommended daily allowances of the vitamins, minerals and trace elements. There is no other single **food** of such low calorific content (411 kcal per day) which achieves this end. It has an enormous potential in preventing malnutrition, particularly in children, pregnant and nursing women and the elderly when used in **addition** to a healthy diet.

Because the Cambridge Diet is very palatable, it is well received by elderly people who very often have problems in chewing food or who become uninterested or too infirm to prepare good, nourishing food. Toddlers often reach a stage of being unconcerned about food and will go for a long time ignoring what is put in front of them. But it has been reported by many counsellors that a child will always want a drink of what he sees his mother drinking. The many varieties of flavours appeal to a child and while he is getting what he thinks is a special grown-up drink, he is in fact, getting much of the nutrition needed in a single milkshake.

## Athletes

It was not long after its introduction in the United States that professional athletes and team players found out the great value of the Cambridge Diet as a nutritional supplement. Among the first to use it were members of the Philadelphia Eagles football team, whose coach, Otto Davis, insisted that all his players should use it regularly as part of their normal training. Some of the benefits claimed were a more sustained energy level during the game and an increased speed of healing of injuries. The early success of the Philadelphia Eagles was so remarkable that many other football teams copied them.

There is another way in which the Cambridge Diet can help sportsmen and women, and that is when they retire. Dennis Franks, a former centre for the Philadelphia Eagles, weighed about 19st (270lb - 122kg), much of which was healthy muscle and important to him as a football player. After retiring from the game, he started the Cambridge Sole Source programme and lost 14lb (6.35kg) in three days and 42lb (19kg) in three weeks. He runs an average of two miles (1.6 km) and does 1 hour of weight lifting per day. Many heavyweight sportsmen die young because after they retire their muscles turn to fat and they do not decrease their body weight to the ideal. It is very important that they should decrease their weight and many of them have found that the use of the Cambridge Diet is a speedy and effective way to do it.

Competitive athletes often have to reduce from 'training weight' to 'performance weight', but need to do so with nutritional assurance. And, of course, they often travel around the world to events where the local diet is not ideal. In these cases, the nutritional supplementation that Cambridge can provide in relatively few calories is ideal.

Nowadays, large numbers of people all around the world regularly use Cambridge as a source of nutrition. They believe it is beneficial, because they feel better, have a higher energy level and have a firm belief that a good nutritional basis can lead to a healthier and longer life.

According to all good nutritional principles, they should be right! They should develop fewer of the diseases of Western-style civilization such as coronary heart disease, cancer and strokes; and because of their lowered metabolism, they should live longer. It is an interesting and important human experiment – and we shall know the answer only in twenty or thirty years from now. I am firmly convinced that they will be proved right.

# The Role of Exercise

7

Very few people can lose weight just by exercise alone. A leading Swedish doctor, who was treating 16 patients with a Cambridge weight loss programme, divided them into two groups. One group had a strenuous workout in the gym three times a week, and the other group just sat down and watched. At the end of three weeks he found there was no difference in weight-loss, even though the exercise group expended 1,650 more calories in physical activity.

To burn up 1lb (450g) of body fat you need to expend about 3,500 calories, so the maximum effect would theoretically be only ½lb (225 g), an amount too small to measure in small groups of people who individually have a wide variation in weight-losses.

This is not to say that I do not feel exercise is important. On the contrary, it is absolutely essential for long term weight maintenance and anyone trying to keep physically fit. Besides slowing down the ageing process, exercise is thought by many doctors to reduce the risk of coronary heart disease.

But there are great dangers in someone undertaking strenuous exercise when they are unused to it. If you are seriously interested, then you should first consult your doctor, especially if you are over the age of forty. He will check that you have no underlying medical condition which contraindicates your starting. Quite a few people have ended up with a coronary attack after strenuous exercise because they were unaware that they had coronary heart disease.

Since overweight people are usually not very keen on exercise and lose weight easily on the diet, they tend to give exercise no further thought. This is a pity because in the long term exercise should be of supreme importance in weight maintenance. The reason for this is that exercise can increase the ratio of muscle to fat in the body. Muscle tissue requires much more energy than fat for maintenance and a person's normal resting metabolism is largely dependent on how much muscle is present in the body. When you exercise, your muscles increase in size and you will continually burn up more energy even when you are not exercising but just sitting still.

If you are following the Cambridge 'Sole Source' programme, it is unlikely that you will build up much muscle, as the number of calories are very restricted. However, on the maintenance plan, when you supplement the diet with additional calories and much more protein, the ratio of muscle to fat will automatically increase, providing that you exercise as well.

In today's fast-paced, quick moving world, many of us find that the greatest amount of exercise we get is what we expend walking from our homes to our cars or the bus. Of course, we do occasionally take the dog for a walk or spend an hour or two swimming while on holiday, but for the most part, we have become much less active than our ancestors, while in fact, still eating more than our bodies need.

If you are very overweight, or have been quite inactive and happen to be over forty, your feelings about exercise might parallel those of a well known comedienne who said, 'The first time I see a jogger smiling, I'll consider trying it,' or another who commented, 'My idea of exercise is a good, brisk sit.' If you have similar feelings, let me encourage you to start exercising; but I suggest you wait until you have been on the Cambridge Diet at least a week before you start. It is important to maintain your new activity levels after you reach your ideal body weight, because it is then that you will reap maximum benefit.

## Types of Exercise

There are many different types of exercise and activity, which can be performed to fulfil different functions. For instance, some activities may be chosen to improve the efficiency of the heart and lungs, others may be used to improve flexibility, and others to increase muscular strength or physical endurance. A well-balanced programme will contain activities that provide a combination of benefits (See box below).

### Fitness Value of Selected Activities

| Exercise | Heart & Lungs | Joint suppleness | Muscle power |
|---|---|---|---|
| Golf (flat course) | ✓ | ✓✓ | ✓ |
| Jogging (brisk) | ✓✓✓✓ | ✓✓ | ✓✓ |
| Swimming | ✓✓✓✓ | ✓✓✓✓ | ✓✓✓✓ |
| Tennis | ✓✓✓ | ✓✓✓ | ✓✓ |
| Walking (brisk) | ✓✓ | ✓ | ✓✓ |

✓✓✓✓ = excellent; ✓✓✓ = good; ✓✓ = fair; ✓ = minimal

(Adapted from 'Complete Family Health Encyclopaedia', British Medical Association; Dorling Kindersley 1996)

### Aerobic exercise –

requires the lungs to take in additional oxygen to meet the requirements of the muscles – the kind of exercise that makes you breathless. Activities such as jogging, rowing, cycling, squash, and swimming fall into this category. Aerobic exercise is the best kind of exercise for improving cardiovascular fitness, and also usually improves the strength and flexibility of certain muscle groups at the same time. For example, jogging improves and strengthens the leg muscles as well as increasing cardiovascular fitness.

## Isometric exercise –

in which one group of muscles exerts pressure against an immovable object (a wall, for example) or against an opposing group of muscles. Although these exercises improve muscle strength, they do not have any effect on cardiovascular fitness or on flexibility because there is no movement involved.

## Isotonic exercise –-

in which the body works against its own weight or against an external weight. Weight-lifting and calisthenics (repetitive exercises that have been designed to stretch and strengthen particular muscle groups) are examples of isotonic exercises.

## Isokinetic exercise –-

combines elements of isometric and isotonic exercise. This is the kind of exercise usually performed on the sophisticated fitness training equipment found in gymnasiums and sports centres.

When exercise is aerobic, large quantities of oxygen are consumed by the muscles and fat, instead of carbohydrate being burned. Thus, aerobics are a great advantage to someone who wants to lose weight, because the body fat is burned in preference to other energy stores. Moreover, body metabolism is speeded up for many hours after a brisk workout.

What exercises are aerobic? Any strenuous, continuous use of your muscles for at least 12 minutes. Thus, swimming, cycling, jogging, walking (for 45 minutes), cross-country skiing, roller and ice skating are all aerobic, providing they are continuous. Other stop-go sports such as tennis, weightlifting, football, golf and other team sports are not aerobic but anaerobic.

What are the further benefits of aerobics? It can do wonders for your heart and lungs and general body metabolism. It produces changes in your brain chemistry which are, in many ways, similar to the benefits of sleeping pills, drugs which lower blood pressure, tranquilizers, antidepressants, without the side effects one normally gets when taking these types of drugs.

I recommend that you practise aerobic exercises at least three times per week (remembering that the critical time for their performance is at least 12 minutes). In the course of time your heart and lungs will benefit by becoming stronger, they will be able to handle more easily a sudden demand for energy without being overworked. The heart rests longer between beats and this is reflected by a drop in pulse rate.

There really is a programme of exercise for everyone who is truly interested in physical fitness. Listed and discussed here are several forms of the most popular exercises available. Exercises for specific parts of the body are not included. If you need special 'toning' exercises you will find many excellent books, articles in magazines and newspapers and literally hundreds of physical fitness centres around the world that can help you tone up where you need it most.

## Swimming

Swimming is a form of exercise for everyone. So if you can't swim, learn now. Swimming offers some unique opportunities to people who, because of age or disability, have not been able to participate in a physical fitness programme before.

Although swimming can be much less strenuous than many other forms of exercise, the results are just as beneficial in improving cardiovascular and muscular endurance, strength and flexibility. Swimming will also provide the same psychological benefits that any other physical activity can provide, but for those people who have not been able to experience a positive fitness programme it opens up a new dimension.

Swimming gives an opportunity to do something well and to enjoy a feeling of success. This is all too often denied to the person with a disability or of advanced age. Being successful at something enhances self image, the sense of achievement and self-esteem.

Swimming is fun, and for persons whose activities are limited, it provides an environment in which frustration may be released safely. To splash, push and kick water is a marvellous release for tension.

Age or physical impairment is far less evident in water. Of those who experience discomfort or inability to walk on land (even those confined to a wheelchair) most will be capable of walking unaided in water. 'The advantage of buoyancy in water makes possible movement which is impossible on land.

Although special programmes may be needed for individuals with severe problems, many persons are indeed able to participate in a regular swimming programme.

Swimming has long been a part of rehabilitation programmes and is now widely used as a relatively painless and yet total physical fitness exercise.

## Jogging and Running

Jogging has become very popular and I have been a keen devotee of it myself. In fact I was one of the first to begin jogging in Cambridge. Back in 1960 1 could be seen jogging along Gog Magog Hills in Cambridge and was even interviewed by a Cambridge newspaper and photographed. I was considered something of a freak. Times have changed!

Those who are physically and mentally up to this form of activity are totally exhilarated by it and converted to it. If, however, you are extremely overweight, your body has to be conditioned beforehand, otherwise it can be very dangerous and can precipitate a heart attack.

This is one of the reasons why it is most important to see your doctor before taking up jogging. Jogging can also cause other problems: tendonitis, inflamed or ruptured Achilles tendons (caused by repeatedly running uphill), sore shins, fractures, and blisters by the thousand.

To help avoid trouble do not wear tight T-shirts which can cause 'jogger's nipple', get a good pair of shoes, and stick to jogging on grass at first.

How do you start a jogging programme? SLOWLY! Take it easy at first, running slowly for 5 minutes, then walk for the same time and repeat until you are comfortably tired. As you become conditioned and the weeks roll by, you can begin to run faster and extend the time, but never attempt more than you feel you can cope with. If you are really interested, consult one of the many books on this form of exercise for a good programme of action. Adopt a running style and have plenty of determination.

Is it worth it? Those who have mastered this form of exercise are extremely enthusiastic and almost fanatical in their praise of it, so much so they become evangelical. They feel a sensible running programme is the *best* way to keep heart and lungs in good condition.

## Gym Exercises and Weight Lifting

Judging by the large number of people who are joining health and fitness centres, gym work-outs and weight lifting seem to fit the needs of many people.

While other will feel it is too strenuous, people who regularly exercise in gyms do develop very efficient cardiovascular systems. The benefits are obvious – having excellent muscle tone, a highly efficient heart, and stronger lungs. Weight lifting is not an aerobic exercise but nevertheless it will build those extra muscles needed to increase your metabolism.

Modern gyms now have trampolines which, besides providing aerobic exercise, are especially beneficial for overweight people, because they alleviate the problem of landing on the ground with too much force. Mini trampolines are also available for those who want to use one in the privacy of their own homes.

Rather surprisingly, working out every day will not give as good results as every other day, especially over a long period of time. All weight-training activities should be supervised by trained personnel, who will ensure you avoid injury and obtain maximum benefit.

## Exercise Machines

All fitness centres and gyms are equipped with a myriad of exercise machines giving a whole range of body trimming exercises for the really enthusiastic fitness convert. For those who prefer to exercise in the privacy of home, there are now many types of multi-gym exercise machines, which are compact and designed to high standards, making them suitable for home use. These machines can be used for a range of exercises and – for those people who find cycling outdoors too dangerous – there are stationary cycling machines for home use.

## Dancing

Ordinary dancing is fun, and aerobic dancing is too! Aerobic dancing is a combination of exercise and dancing and is a complete physical fitness programme. This is your opportunity to express yourself physically to music by laughing, yelling, jumping, kicking, jogging, stretching, sliding and swinging.

Judging by the overflowing classes that are springing up everywhere – such as line-dancing, ceroc, salsa etc – aerobic dancing has become a sensation, especially for women. And although aerobic dancing classes are quite popular it is not necessary to join a class to enjoy its benefits. No great skill or technique is required. There are literally hundreds of books, tapes and records to help you learn it at home.

As with other forms of exercise mentioned here, I would suggest that you seek expert advice, and start very slowly. To reap full benefit, aerobic dancing should be done a minimum of three times weekly.

## Cycling

Cycling is unique among popular fitness programmes in that it does *not* take weeks for a beginner to build up a gradual exercise plan.

If, however, you have previously been a sedentary person, a little sensible caution is advisable. For those over the age of thirty-five and who are a bit out of shape, or those who suffer from a heart, lung or circulatory disease, it would be best to see a physician to determine your level of fitness before starting.

Most of us have grown up as cyclists but gave it up after leaving school. Cars and sitting in front of television sets have greatly affected this once totally normal form of exercise. As a boy growing up in East Anglia I travelled extensively all over Europe, often cycling over 100 miles (161 km)a day. Lack of time and my hectic schedule have almost put a complete stop to the cycling I am able to do.

Cycling is a marvellous way to attain a heart rate that expands the blood flow to the muscles and increases the lung's capacity to absorb oxygen, thus avoiding heart and lung disease. So much is offered to the cyclist; freedom to exercise whenever the urge strikes, an opportunity to get out into fresh air, and economical transportation.

I would give just one caution about cycling: learn how to ride safely. Obtain a manual of bicycle safety rules and become a sensible, safe cyclist. Not every city has the same problem that exists here in Cambridge (20,000 students and 19,000 of them use cycles), but an irresponsible cyclist runs the risk of not living long enough to reach the goal of being physically fit!

## Walking

It has been said that walking is the safest and most efficient form of exercise. Merely increasing the amount of daily walking can give great benefits. You actually do *not* need to worry about technique or exercise regimen – just wear comfortable shoes and begin the walking habit.

I have long been accused by my family and friends of walking them to exhaustion! I enjoy walking and walking with speed and vigour and I personally find walking most efficient for improving overall fitness. It uses more muscles in a continuous uniform action than most other terms of exercise and it remains accessible to you throughout your lifetime.

Walking has become the most often used medical programme to prevent heart related diseases and to rehabilitate those who have been stricken with heart trouble. There are approximately four basic forms used in walking programmes:

☐ **Strolling** – the slowest form of walking, but just as significant in results, because the repetitious movements of the body's walking muscle groups aid circulation and helps to burn off some calories (at a very slow rate, of course).

☐ **Normal** – normal walking is usually considered an average speed of three mph, and can be used as a fitness programme simply by doing more of it by walking to work; using the stairs instead of the lift; taking a walk during coffee break; taking a walk after meals; taking a walk before a meal can actually *depress* your appetite

☐ **Aerobic Walking** – is any style of walking done with speed and consists of sustained rapid breathing while vigorously moving your arms and legs. Try it for between 15 and 30 minutes, three times per week. Just maintain a brisk pace. As you become more physically fit you can speed up and extend your time, helping to continue making progress.

☐ **Long Distance** – is for people who really enjoy walking and are physically fit.

## To Exercise or Not

Reading this chapter may have made you so physically tired that any thoughts of taking up exercise may have already evaporated! The benefits of increased activity levels include being physically fit and healthy. Whether you take up an organised activity or simply increase the amount of walking you do, it is important that you enjoy it! Experiment with local clubs and find out for yourself what type of exercise you think you would like doing best. In the long term you will only persist if it gives you pleasure.

## Using exercise to burn calories

Healthy exercise has always been part of the Cambridge programme, but trying to assess the effect of exercise is not always easy, because the number of calories you burn depends upon your weight and the type and intensity of the activity.

The table overleaf gives an indication of calories you could expect to burn in 30 minutes in a range of everyday activities. The rates are based on two nominal weights, and the table has been compiled from a number of sources found on the Internet.

Obviously, if you exercise at a higher intensity level, you will be working harder, expending more energy and burning more calories than someone who is not working quite so hard.

## Burning Calories

*The figures given below show the approximate numbers of calories you might expect to lose in 30 minutes of these everyday activities*

| Activity | 9st 9lb (61kg) | 12st 12lb (82kg) |
|---|---|---|
| Aerobic (high) | 275 | 369 |
| Aerobic (moderate) | 165 | 222 |
| Basketball | 256 | 345 |
| Bowling | 40 | 57 |
| Cycling | 180 | 288 |
| Dancing – actively | 150 | 200 |
| Football | 240 | 320 |
| Gardening | 140 | 190 |
| Golf | 147 | 200 |
| Hiking | 150 | 200 |
| Housework – cleaning | 190 | 270 |
| Jogging | 320 | 440 |
| Racquetball | 240 | 330 |
| Rowing | 196 | 260 |
| Running | 360 | 480 |
| Shopping | 110 | 150 |
| Sitting | 35 | 51 |
| Standing | 68 | 95 |
| Swimming | 250 | 348 |
| Tennis | 200 | 268 |
| Volleyball | 88 | 120 |
| Walking | 130 | 175 |
| Walking upstairs | 280 | 370 |

# The End Result

*8*

## The Last Few Pounds/Kilos

It is a common experience for some people to plateau just short of their target weight. Many of them start off following the Cambridge Diet correctly and quickly experience dramatic results. They begin to look and feel better and are proud of their progress. Their friends notice how slim they are looking and ask what was the reason for their success.

Then something very curious happens. Just when they are about to get down to their ideal weight, they either plateau or put weight on, which means that they are not following their diet programme as they should. Often they make excuses, claiming to be a victim of a bad cold or of being depressed. One psychologist suggests that the reason is that some people are fearful of achieving their goal – ideal weight-loss. If they were to achieve it there would be no further challenges for them.

On the other hand, it could be explained by a loss of motivation. One lady, who had been severely overweight and successfully shed much of the excess, could see what tremendous progress she had made whenever she looked at her 'before' photographs. Then, someone she hadn't seen for a long time came along and went into raptures about how much she had changed and how wonderful she looked. As a result, a sense of self-satisfaction settled in and that was the end of her desire and motivation to continue to lose weight.

Whatever the explanation, everyone is unanimous that the last few pounds/kilos are certainly the hardest!

## Is it Worthwhile?

If you are severely overweight and have lost pounds and pounds to achieve your ideal weight, you will have found the going tough. While the Cambridge programmes are easy to use and a sure way of achieving success, you will need strong motivation and a lot of grit and determination to continue month after month.

For those who were moderately overweight or had just a small amount to lose it was easier, but still required a high degree of motivation. Was all the trouble worth it? And will the long-term benefits be easily apparent? Let's look at some of the positive benefits you will achieve:

☐ There is a feeling of great achievement to have solved finally what for many years has been an extremely difficult problem. Many of the emotional and physical problems caused by that excess weight will have disappeared, one hopes, for ever.

☐ From a medical viewpoint, you are almost certain to live longer. Your risk of coronary heart disease, diabetes, or high blood pressure are very much reduced because you have reached a normal, healthy weight.

☐ If you have been suffering with any of these diseases, the symptoms may have been very much improved by your weight-loss. The chances are that you will be able to live a longer and healthier life.

☐ From the physical viewpoint, you will feel much better. You will sleep less, be more active and athletic and have a greater zest for living life to its fullest.

☐ You will be astonished at how youthful and attractive you look. Your friends and relatives will comment on it. You will be able to dress in more stylish clothes and have a very much improved body image.

☐ Your social life will be improved. Instead of avoiding people, you will make an increasing circle of new friends and acquaintances, purely because you are not hiding yourself away from life and public gaze.

☐ You will be much better off financially, too. Fewer days off work because of illness, the continual taking of the Cambridge Diet as a nutritional supplement will ensure that you feel well, are able to work harder and thus have better prospects of earning more.

*From every point of view it is well worth it!!*

# Part Two – The Cambridge Success

# Weight Loss Success Stories

**9**

## Alison Walter
### Evesham, England

Until recently, Alison Walter had been overweight for as long as she could remember. Over the years, Alison had tried diet after diet, but despite the occasional short-term success, she was unable to keep the weight off. By April 2002, her weight had risen to 20st (280lb - 127kg). Something had to be done.

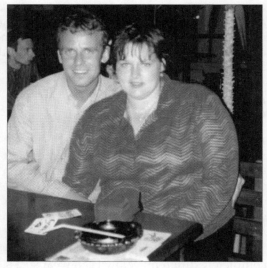

"I was at my lowest weight for years when I met my fiancee in 1996," remembers Alison. "But within 18 months I had regained about 5 stone and as a result became very unhappy – longing to be slim and 'normal' like my friends. In April 2001, I got pregnant and although the pregnancy was quite a healthy one, towards the end my blood pressure became raised and carrying a baby plus 9 stone extra weight I was extremely uncomfortable.

"It was at this point that I decided that once the baby was born I was going to diet – I never wanted to feel like that again. Thomas was born in January, so it was now time to start shedding those excess pounds. I didn't want Thomas to have a 'fat' mummy; I wanted to be able to run around with him, take him swimming. All the things I wouldn't have been able to do when carrying the unwanted weight. I knew what I should have been eating, but I was fairly inactive for about 8 weeks after the birth and it was all too easy to turn to those high-calorie snacks during the day while I was alone with Thomas. It felt like I would never be able to stick to a diet and the more unhappy I became about it, the more I ate!

The turning point for Alison came when a friend visited and told her about a Diet which had helped a friend lose a lot of weight in a short space of time. "This is how I discovered the Cambridge Diet," says Alison. "I found the

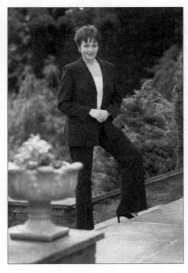

number of Daphne Richards, who was my local Counsellor. After I arranged to see her I have not looked back since!"

Alison found the Sole Source programme very straightforward, and the pounds just fell away. Cambridge allows people to eliminate food completely. "For the first time in years, I didn't spend every waking moment thinking about what my next meal or snack would be," says Alison, who lost over 7stone in seven months with Cambridge.

"I have obviously changed physically, but the big change has been psychological," says Alison. "I am so much more confident. I don't feel like a second-class citizen any more, and I can hold my head high when I walk into public places, instead of wanting to fade away into the background. My family are really proud of me, especially my fiancée Dave, who has supported me all the way through. We are now planning our wedding and I am looking forward to being able to wear a wonderful dress and look back at the photos to see a slim, happy person instead of an overweight, unhappy one! Thank you, Cambridge, but thanks especially to Daphne Richards, my counsellor, for all her support, kindness and friendship over the last seven months."

## Ajit Singh
## 49-year old from Singapore

Ajit Singh used to be so obese that he could not fit into an airline seat. Once, on the flight to Kuching, he had to sit at the front portion of the plane, a 737, as he could not buckle up on a normal seat. His Sikh bangle got stuck on his wrist as he grew fatter, and his watch had to have an extension strap.

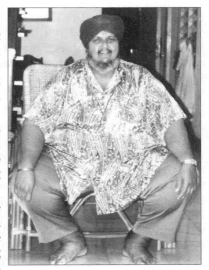

But now, life for the 49-year old is completely different: "Now I can wear socks! I couldn't before because my feet were too swollen. And I can wear my engagement ring for the first time in 20 years."

Ajit had been piling on the pounds since he was 30. He had tried a few diets, even appetite suppressants, but they did more harm than good. When he stopped taking them, he gained even more weight. By 1998, his weight had soared to 34st 11lb (487lb - 221kg) when he started taking the Cambridge Diet. After a year on Cambridge, his weight is a much healthier 21st 4lb (298lb - 135kg).

"I lost 8kg within 10 days on the Sole Source Diet," says Ajit, "and I felt much lighter, more energetic and happier. After 2 to 3 weeks on the Diet, you don't get any food cravings," he said, "even if meals are on the table."

Ajit used to refuse to even go shopping with his family, but after two months on the Diet, he travelled to Singapore! Nowadays, Ajit is much more mobile, and is delirious with joy for being able to travel on a bus.

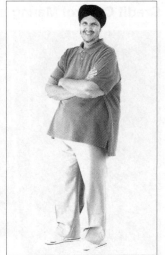

"I am buying different clothes," says Ajit, "and when my friends saw me in a T-shirt, I was the talk of the town!

In common with other who have lost weight, the benefits are not just external, because Ajit's health has also improved: "I used to have dark patches on my skin, but all that has cleared up since I started on the Cambridge Diet. There were marks round my neck and these have disappeared too. I think it is the "pure food" in the Cambridge Diet." But the best gift from Cambridge, he reckons, is that his thyroid is functioning normally again after being hypothyroid for so long.

Ajit is still on Cambridge as he hopes to lose another 14 to 16 kg to maintain his weight at 120kg, which is ideal for his height of 6ft 2".

## Cory Hipolito
## 53-year old senior manager from Manila, Philippines

"I started to realise I was getting overweight in 1996. My daughter is so beautiful and I remembered that I used to be the same slim shape she is. Wanting to look my best was my primary concern, although I also realised from my experience in the insurance industry that being overweight may affect my health later in life.

"I started taking the Cambridge Diet in early 2002 when I weighted 11$^{st}$ (154lb - 69.9kg). I took it to replace two meals a day. My counsellor taught me to be aware of the calories I was taking in and of what foods contained the most and least calories. She also made me aware of which foods gave me the nutrients my body needs.

"After the first month, I had lost 17 pounds, and in total I lost 24 pounds before I went onto a weight maintenance programme. The first things people said when they saw I had lost weight were that I looked younger and that my face did not sag in the way they had seen on people who had lost weight using other methods. What they can't see are the changes inside me. I feel healthier; my blood pressure has stabilized; my bad cholesterol is way down and my good cholesterol is up. Added to this, I am so happy when people say my daughter looks so much like me.

"I have recommended the Cambridge Diet to a lot of my friends. I guess my referrals have helped my counsellor get quite rich!

"One of the things I have noticed is that those who take weight loss seriously succeed. Those who think the weight will just disappear without having to try get nowhere. At least if you use the Cambridge way, you know you are doing your body no harm."

## Roy Fuller
### Credit Control Manager from Milton Keynes, England

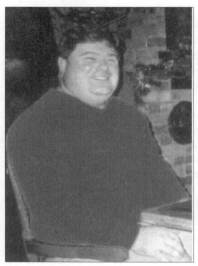

Roy Fuller is no stranger to losing weight. He has tried a number of diets over the years, but in a familiar sounding tale, his successes were never maintained: after dropping weight, he would soon find himself rebounding to an even greater weight. But March 2001 was a turning point for Roy because he was horrified to discover he weighed 26st (364lb - 165kg). He was determined to lose weight - and maintain it this time.

He turned to Sylvia Dennis (a Counsellor since 1986) who regularly ran "Men Only" groups of Cambridge Dieters in Milton Keynes. "The group situation worked well for me," Roy remembers, "and the weight soon started tumbling off. After a few months I had lost nearly 10 stone, and I was determined not to rebound this time."

Thanks to Sylvia's support and encouragement he added sensible food choices to his menus, and by following the recommended maintenance programme, the weight continued to reduce.

"I benefited enormously from losing weight, and not just because I was more mobile. This achievement has given me more self-esteem, and I have much more confidence in all aspects of my life. People no longer judge me because I couldn't control my weight. All of my work colleagues could see the improvement, and were impressed enough to want to try the Cambridge Diet for themselves. With Sylvia's encouragement, I decided to become a Counsellor in my own right. Sylvia helped me complete the training and accreditation. I have over 30 customers, all of whom are achieving dramatic results themselves.

Roy gets a buzz at the prospect of helping other people and he organised a number of events for the 'BBC Children in Need' charity appeal, raising over £900 through sponsorship

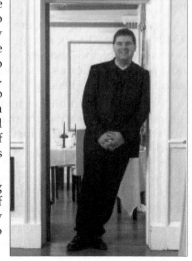

and a 'Guess the Weight' competition. Roy was one of the 'Slimmers of the Year' in 2001.

"I look and feel 10 years younger and am happy to support and advise others who decide that they don't want to be fat or obese any more. Thanks to the Cambridge Diet, I have been given another chance to reclaim my wasted years."

## Cik Fazrin Audra
### 29-year old mother of 4, Malaysia

"After I delivered my third child, my weight was at 11st 7lb (161lb - 73 kg). But, when I was pregnant with my fourth, my weight had gone up by 20 kilogrammes and although I lost some weight after giving birth, after 2 months of confinement, my weight was still 13st 5lb (187lb - 85 kg).

"One of my friends recommended me to try The Cambridge Diet. My husband supported me and we both tried Cambridge for one week. I lost 3.5 kg and my husband lost 5 kg. We continued to take Cambridge Diet meals for another two weeks with 3 meals replacement and I lost another 8 kg. I slowly reduced it with 3 meals for one day and four days with 2 meals replacement until I reached 10st 3lb (143lb - 65 kg).

"And now I really believe that by replacing your normal meal with The Cambridge Diet, it was the fastest, healthier and effective way to reduce weight. Thank you The Cambridge Diet."

## Ms Priscilla Ng
### Marketing Executive, Malaysia

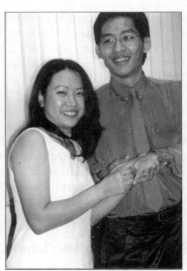

"I wanted to be one of the most beautiful brides for my coming wedding ceremony but with my body shape, I did not have the confidence to try on my wedding gown. But, thanks to my best

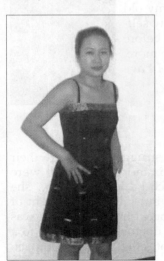

friend - who recommended me to try the Cambridge Diet - I lost 4 kg in the first three days by taking a Cambridge meal 3 times a day in place of an ordinary meal.

"That really inspired me to continue in getting down to my ideal weight. After all, it did not have the "yo-yo effect" even though I stopped for one week. In fact, I still managed to maintain my new weight!! I have the confidence towards the Cambridge Diet - because it works."

## Nilgun Okmen
## Turkey

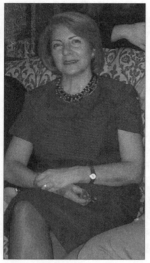

"I was very interested in becoming a distributor for Cambridge in Turkey. But, first of all, I wanted to test this diet program on myself. I did have some extra kilos but I hadn't bothered about it too much. I wanted to feel the hunger, to examine the side effects of the 'Sole Source' programme diet before recommending it to other people.

"In preparation, I started with 'Step2 (790kcal)' for 3 days. Then, I continued with the 'Sole Source' programme. After 10 days, I had lost 4kg. I thought it was miraculous. On 'Sole Source', I had 3 sachets of soup or drink, plus one meal bar that I divided in two; I ate the first half at 5 o'clock and saved the second half for 10 pm.

"Despite drinking 2.5 ltr of water a day, I still felt hungry for almost 10 days. I was consuming an extra meal by eating a meal bar, but I didn't want to give up because chewing made me happy.

"After the loss of 4 kg, I stopped weighing myself, and I started to walk 40 minutes every day. I augmented my physical exercises such as 30 minutes swimming four times a week, 40 minutes walking every day and 1 hour aerobic twice a week. After two weeks, I tried the 'add a meal' week, and then followed the Step 2 programme for a week, and then the Step 3 (1000 kcal) programme. At the end of six weeks I had lost 6kg.

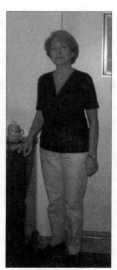

"I feel myself very fit and very energetic, and the people around me are astonished at my loss of weight in so short a time. They want to buy CD soups. Now I can use my old clothes that I couldn't use for four years. I gained my self-confidence, and I bought a bikini! I'm healthier. than before because I have changed my style of living: I exercise more, and I eat less - and I know how to lose weight. I have Cambridge as a fuse!

## Jayne Redman
## Post-office worker; Leeds, England

Most people can recall a defining moment in their struggle to manage their weight. In Jayne's case the words: 'This woman is morbidly obese' were horrifying. "For the first time, it hit home how much I'd let myself go," she remembers. "I was just under 17st (238lb - 108kg), but I'd never thought of myself as obese." Struggling with a long-running back problem, which was aggravated by her size, Jayne had gone to see her doctor for a referral to a specialist. It was the doctor's words in his referral notes that made the impact.

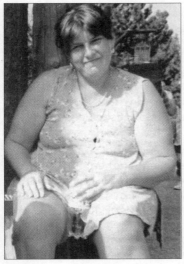

"I knew I was fat," says Jayne, "but always thought it was in control; losing and gaining anything between three and four stone over the years. When David and I got married 14 years ago, I was down to 11st (69.8kg), but after the kids came along, I just grew."

Jayne had tried varied slimming clubs without success, so she was skeptical about signing up for another one — and doubtful about her ability to go it alone. But, whilst working as a manicurist in a friend's beauty salon, Jayne noticed one of her regular clients getting slimmer by the week. Eventually, Jayne got the details of a local diet club, and decided to start immediately after her wedding anniversary. So, in July 2001, she had her first one-to-one consultation with Counsellor Carol Lyons.

"Carol said that I'd start off on three Cambridge meals a day for the first month. Then I could choose a proper meal from the Cambridge menu planner to supplement the Cambridge meals. The first few days were difficult because I was starving, and by the third day had a bad headache." But Carol reassured her that these short-term effects were normal, and sure enough, after the first week, the cravings and hunger pangs subsided.

"The great thing for me was not having to think about what I was eating," says Jayne. "My family and friends all supported me all the way as well." says Jayne. The weight fell away: 4st in 4 months and by July of 2002 - almost exactly a year since she started - Jayne reached her target weight and stabilised at a healthy 9st (57kg) — a loss of about 8 st, nearly half her original weight.

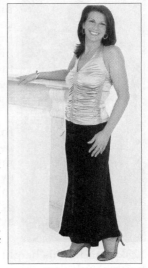

After winning her battle of the bulge, Jayne is determined not to slip back into her old habits, and she still uses Cambridge for nutrition and continues to see Carol twice a month. Jayne's family — husband David and children, James and Holly — are still getting used to their new-look wife and mother. Young Holly wanted to know how to spell 'thin' for a story she was writing about her mummy at school, whilst David had a willing partner on a charity-sponsored walk, trekking 43 miles over the North Yorkshire Moors. "It was exhausting," Jayne remembers, "but I was proud of myself."

## Wong Yuk Lin
## Production Supervisor from New Territories, Hong Kong

Wong Yuk Lin started to use the Cambridge Diet in November 2002. At the age of 50 and with a weight of 10st 4lb (144lb - 65.3kg), she was beginning to have concerns about her health. In particular, she knew that her weight was causing her to feel pain in her knees and made her short of breath when climbing stairs. She spoke to a Cambridge Diet counsellor and decided that she needed to lose 15lb (6.8kg). This she achieved quite quickly.

"I was so happy with the results. At first, my friends and family doubted that the Diet would work. Some of my colleagues even laughed at me when I sat down with a soup while they enjoyed their rice at lunchtime. I only weighed myself once each week and was always so happy to see how well I was doing. This really gave me the motivation to carry on. When I got down to 9st 3lb (129 lb - 58.5kg), I no longer had pains in my knees and I felt so much lighter and more energetic. But, there were even more benefits to my Diet than I was expecting. My skin looks so much better now - more shiny. Some say it looks younger! And, as well as this, my digestive system has improved."

In order to keep her weight down, she still uses the Cambridge Diet to replace one meal each day. "I'm proud to tell people I used the Cambridge Diet. I certainly don't keep it a secret!"

## Sylwek
## 22-year old student from Wloclawek, Poland

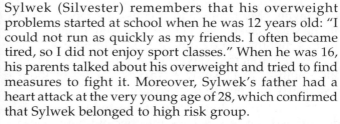

Sylwek (Silvester) remembers that his overweight problems started at school when he was 12 years old: "I could not run as quickly as my friends. I often became tired, so I did not enjoy sport classes." When he was 16, his parents talked about his overweight and tried to find measures to fight it. Moreover, Sylwek's father had a heart attack at the very young age of 28, which confirmed that Sylwek belonged to high risk group.

So, he started to observe the rules of proper nutrition, following a diet for youngsters. His mother was in permanent contact with dietician to determine his daily menus. It was effective during a school year, when everything was monitored by his mother and he was able to lose a few kilos. But during summer vacation, after getting fast food, chips, Coke etc, the weight would rise again.

When he was 21, Sylwek weighed 19st 5lb (271lb - 123kg) and at his height of 5ft 11in (1.80m), he was 40kg overweight. He had trouble with sleep, high blood pressure and high cholesterol levels. He has had a detailed medical check every year, so he realised that each kilogram more has had a detrimental influence on his health status. Something had to change.

"Lake yachting is my hobby. I noticed that one of my friends had lost 20 kg in weight - and during the next season, he maintained this weight. I asked him how he had done this, and he mentioned the name of the Cambridge Diet. I then found out that my dietician was a Cambridge Counsellor, but she could not offer it to me earlier, as I was too young to use it."

After studying the programme in detail, Sylwek decided to follow it for 3 weeks on 'Sole Source' and then 3 weeks maintenance. Today his weight is 14st 14lb (200lb - 91kg) and this year even the summer vacation did not increase his weight: no chips, but low calories crispies; no french fries but fresh fruit and vegetables; no Coke, but mineral water.

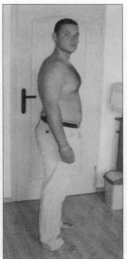

"I would like to lose another 5 kg and believes absolutely in my success with Cambridge. Losing weight is very difficult, but after that it is necessary to change nutrition habits to avoid the 'yo-yo' effect. I realise that a proper diet, combined with physical exercise, will offer much better results in weight loss. These days, I visit the swimming pool and fitness club quite often, going there on a bicycle."

Teresa, his counsellor, comments: "Sylwek could thank his parents for his health and lost kilograms. It is due to their rationality and dedication to fight for his success. They strongly have supported him in his obesity fight and now in changing his nutrition habits. I think today they all have already succeeded."

## Wong Kam Ying
## Fanling, Hong Kong

Wong Kam Ying's weight had been increasing steadily for a number of years, but she didn't really trust any diet products.

"You always see them on the TV and in the newspaper being promoted by some beautiful starlet and I thought they didn't look believable. One of my friends had used the Cambridge Diet many years before. I still didn't know whether I would buy it, but she told me that she had been successful because of the Cambridge counsellor's support. So, I gave a call and was very impressed by the counsellor from the beginning. She told me what I needed to do and told me why people succeed and fail when it comes to dieting and keeping the weight off. She was very honest and I trusted her.

"I started off on 'Sole Source', then moved onto replacing two meals. Within three weeks, I'd lost 18lb (8kg). I felt so much lighter and healthier. My counsellor was always on the telephone encouraging me. At times, I felt she was more proud of my weight loss than I was! When I got down to 9st 8lb (134lb - 60.8kg) - a loss of 24lb - my counsellor and I decided that I should start to maintain that weight. I've been at that weight ever since, still using one sachet each day for lunch.

"I really thought taking a Diet would make me feel bad. Looking back, I can only think how happy the Cambridge Diet has made me feel."

## Marion Cutts
## Sheffield, England

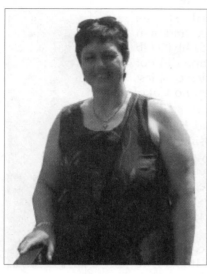

After years of 'yo-yo' dieting, Marion had resigned herself to staying overweight: "I was so disillusioned, I believed I should accept myself as I was. I loved clothes but I just had to wear whatever I could get into. My dream was to wear jeans and to look my age.

But in 2000, Marion was confined to bed with intense back pain which made her realise that the time had come to tackle her weight problem. "I joined forces with one of my neighbours and soon realised that her weight was dropping far more quickly than mine and she had so much more energy! When she told me that she was using the Cambridge Diet, at first I felt a little nervous of a new dieting method, but I spent a week reading the background to the Diet and wrestling with my apprehension. But Sheila Briggs - who became my Counsellor — understood my feelings very quickly and told me that it was not compulsory: that it was my choice. Sheila understood me and realised that I needed to retain my independence. So I chose to take what I had always wanted and I haven't looked back."

Within 5 months, Marion's weight had gone from 17st 4lb (242lb - 109.8kg) down to 12st 11lb179lb- 81.1kg). Marion says: "I was thrilled with my new size and eventually plucked up courage to go into an exclusive dress shop with my mother. There, on the rail, was the dress of my dreams and I couldn't resist trying it on. Imagine my feelings when the dress fitted perfectly and it was a size 14. Needless to say, I just had to buy it!"

But Marion did not just benefit from new clothes: when Marion returned to her Consultant to discuss the terrible back pain she had suffered, his response was 'well done, you have cured yourself, keep up the good work!'

Over a year after he dramatic weight loss, Marion is maintaining her new shape: "I don't comfort eat any more," she says. "I feel happy with my weight now, and Cambridge suits me so well and works much better than a food-based diet. I always have a hot chocolate for breakfast and regularly have a bar for lunch. I eat more protein and plenty of fruit, so I feel so much healthier now.

## Martyn Barrett
## 55-year old Company director, Amersfoort, Holland

"Not everyone is lucky enough to get a second chance and I consider myself very fortunate. Not only to have found the Cambridge Diet again for myself, but also to be given the chance to introduce it into Holland." So says Martyn Barratt, once a man of 26st (384lb - 165kg) who now weighs 14st (196lb - 90kg), and determined to keep it that way with the help of his partner in life and business — Patricia McGraw.

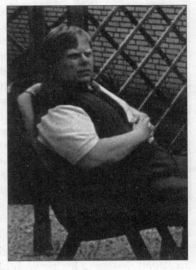

Martyn calls himself "an emotional eater" because he was not encouraged to show his emotions: "I would eat when I was happy and eat when I was depressed," he remembers. "Like most other 'fat' people, I also used to convince myself that I didn't have a problem." However, despite trying a continuous stream of diets his weight continued to rise. Moving to the Netherlands in 1974 made matters worse and boosted his weight to a staggering 165 kg. But in 1985, on returning to England to see his dying father, a nurse told him about the Cambridge Diet, and in fifteen months he was down from 26 to 12 and a half stone.

"For the first time in my life I was really happy with myself and much more self confident. For twelve months I kept my weight down by using the Cambridge Diet as a regular part of my maintenance programme."

But, unfortunately, the next five years were extremely hard, and included the break-up of Martyn's marriage. "One of the main reasons was that our relationship was unable to cope with the change in me since I lost the weight," he says, "and gradually I returned to old bad habits — eating to suppress my emotions.

"Then I met Patricia," remembers Martyn. "Within a few months, she had turned my life around completely. She had lost over 40kg since being in Holland and appreciated what I had gone through. With her help and patience I was able to stabilize my weight at around 145 kg and — in September 1995 whilst we were in England visiting my family — I saw an advertisement for the Cambridge Diet. This started me thinking seriously again about dieting. After a further two months, I felt I was mentally ready to start. My weight was 147 kg when I contacted Counsellor Carol Needham.".

"With lots of support from her, I finally reached my target weight of 14st 2lb (198lb - 90kg)," Martyn says. "Since then I have been using the Cambridge Diet on a regular basis to try and keep my weight under control."

77

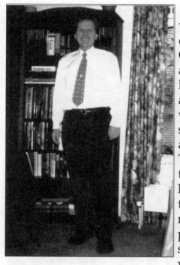

But Cambridge did more than change his weight, it drastically changed his life! Martyn continues: "I was very enthusiastic about Cambridge the first time, and had made enquiries about distributing the diet in Holland. Ten years later - and still as enthusiastic - I enquired again and was delighted to find that Cambridge Export were looking for a distributor there. Holland is similar to other countries in terms of overweight, and it was time for me to seek a new career move. Ten years after I first had the dream I was offered the chance to make it reality. Both Patricia and I have both experienced the heartbreak and pain that being fat can bring and Holland has a huge number and variety of so-called "slimming" products on the market, most of which only succeed in increasing that heartbreak. Together with the Cambridge Diet we are slowly changing all that.

"In Holland, VLCD's are accepted by most nutritional authorities as being an effective way of losing weight for really overweight people. With the weight maintenance guidance provided by a trained Cambridge Counsellor, it is one of the most effective ways to encourage people to change their eating habits. If, by bringing Cambridge to Holland — and by sharing our own experiences — we can succeed in helping just a small proportion of the overweight people in Holland to lose weight, then our own dream will also be fulfilled. Not everyone is lucky enough to get a second chance. I consider myself extremely lucky, not only to have found the Cambridge Diet again for myself, but also to be given the chance to help others by introducing it into Holland. The Cambridge Diet is my very own miracle."

## Joyce Ongpauco
## 28-year old from Alabang, Philippines

Joyce became overweight after giving birth to her second child. She had put on 25lb (11.3kg) and could not get them off again.

"I tried going to the gym but it didn't work for me. Every time I looked at the scales, there didn't seem to have been any change at all, despite all the effort I felt I was putting in. Then I made a big mistake. I bought some 'Bangkok' pills. These are pills smuggled in from other countries which I now know are not at all safe. They contain Phen-phen and no one had warned me about the possible effects of this on me. I had terrible palpitations and great difficulty sleeping. My heart beat became irregular too.

"My family were so worried when I told them I wanted to try the Cambridge Diet. They thought I might get sick again. But I knew I had to lose weight. I felt so sad that I couldn't get back to my old shape. I love parties, so it was depressing for me not to be enthusiastic when I was going out with my family and friends. With the Cambridge Diet, it is very easy to lose weight. All you need is discipline and the help of your counsellor. Having someone always there to help and guide you is great. It's like a having a second mum to praise and discipline you. I have the three most powerful tools in making my weight loss a success. I have the Cambridge Diet. I have my counsellor and I have my determination to lose weight so that I can feel good about myself."

Joyce is now back to her target weight of 8st 8lb (120lb - 54.4kg) and maintaining that weight by using the Cambridge Diet.

# Teresa
# Warsaw, Poland

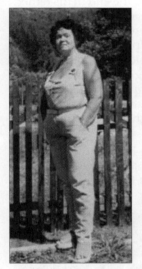

After she retired, Teresa found that her weight increased by to 12st 8lb (176lb - 80kg). A slower pace of life rate, fewer resposibilities - and pleasure in eating were the reasons. She did not feel well, when observing good-looking slim friends. One of her friends recommended her to use the Cambridge Diet.

"It was not an easy decision, and especially starting the programme was very difficult. The first success reached after 3-weeks on Sole Source increased my self-confidence and pushed me further." Over a period of 4 months, Teresa followed 'Sole Source' for 3 weeks and then Step 2 (2 sachets of Cambridge plus 1 'normal' meal) for the next 3 weeks; then repeat.

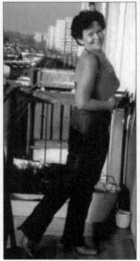

"Each day I felt better; I was lighter and more efficient. My medical check confirmed a decrease of cholesterol level. I have lost not only kilograms but years as well i.e. I feel younger today than before.

"I have learnt to live a different way and decided to help others. I have joined the Cambridge family and become a Counsellor. I am very reliable to my patrons, showing them my old photos and giving them advice based on my own experience. I have changed all my clothing. Today, I am 66 years old and my weight has dropped to 9st 5lb (131lb - 59.5kg) and my way of nutrition is absolutely changed. I am fully satisfied with each person that lost weight with Cambridge under my supervision, and can look in the mirror today with a clear conscience."

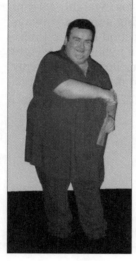

### Paul Carney
### Leisure operative from Castlebar, Eire

Paul Carney is only half the man he used to be. This time last year, Paul, weighed just under 24 stone (nearly 150 kg) before he started a weight loss programme with Cambridge Health Plan, which has helped him to shed nearly 10 stone (60 kgs) - over 40 percent of his original weight. His successful weight loss has earned him the title of Cambridge's 'Slimmer of the Year' in 2002.

By March 2002, Paul had reached the end of his tether: "I knew that my weight was a major problem," he remembers. "My eating habits were out of control and working behind the bar didn't help." He was very self-conscious about his size and considered quitting work completely. His sister Bernie suggested he tried the Cambridge Diet and his doctor supported the idea. With the help of his Cambridge Counsellor, Anne Tobin, he managed to get through the first difficult month and then found that the rapid weight loss he experienced just encouraged him to maintain the Diet.

The big change came after a couple of months when he began to increase his activity levels. "I started walking - and felt fantastic. Before the diet, walking was too uncomfortable. My feet used to swell and I could barely walk at all," says Paul, who now walks up to 5 miles a day with ease.

The transformation is remarkable and Paul still gets a buzz when an old customer from the bar asks him what happened to the big barman! But it is the huge increase in Paul's self-confidence which is the most dramatic change. Whereas before he was reluctant to go out in public, the new slim-line Paul thoroughly enjoyed his prize-winning visit to Norwich - which involved his first ever flight - for a new outfit and a professional photo shoot. And he also enjoyed local celebrity status recently when he was invited to referee an exhibition snooker match between Jimmy White and Tony Drago.

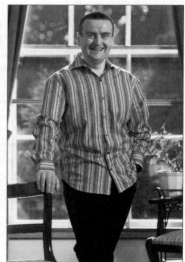

The best news is that - several months after reaching his target weight of 14st (196lb - 88.9kg) - he has maintained his weight loss. "Cambridge has helped me understand the importance of correct nutrition and healthy eating," says Paul, "and I am extremely happy with the new me!"

## Jane Dart
## Wolverhampton, England

When Jane first entered the Wolverhampton Diet Centre in August 1988, it was a case of 'it's now or never'. She was the heaviest she had ever been, and was looking for a diet that was fast, safe and easy with no calorie counting or weighing and measuring of food. "I sat down nervously," says Jane, "a typical overweight, under-confident lady of 12 st 9 lb (80kg). But, after talking with my Counsellor, Helen Gardiner, it became apparent that Cambridge was the diet I had been looking for. After seeing my doctor to obtain his signature I began the Diet three days later.

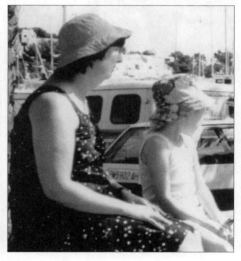

"As an ex-Maths teacher, I was used to doing things by the rules and I approached the Diet with the same precision. I stuck to it religiously — the only exception being a glass of free champagne on a weekend break — and I kept meticulous records of my progress."

Cambridge seemed to suit her perfectly and — with lots of support and encouragement from Helen — Jane reached her initial target of 10st (63.5kg) in three months. "I felt so well that I then decided to aim for 9st 2lb(58kg) — the advised target on the height / weight chart. For the first time in many years, my confidence returned. No longer was I the shrinking violet in the corner, always at the back in photographs (or preferably not there at all). Instead, when at the last minute I was asked to step in as a model at a fashion show at my daughter's school, I was happy to be on the catwalk for all to see! Only someone who has been overweight, as I had been, can appreciate how I felt at that moment.

"With my new found confidence and figure, fashionable clothes started to appeal to me. Trying on a size 12 after having to buy elasticated size 16s was a big thrill! Helen often came shopping with me and encouraged me to buy clothes and wear make-up."

However, the 'new' Jane did not stop there, because activity and exercise was next on the agenda. Gradually increasing her activity levels, Jane now has a regular weekly aerobics class and was invited to be part of a fitness and aerobics display team.

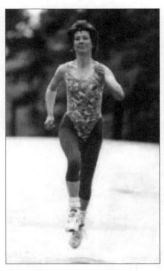

"Before losing weight, I frequently ate between meals and was very inactive. But now, my attitude to food has changed. I now eat much more healthily. I enjoy a Cambridge meal bar with two glasses of water, followed by a banana for lunch and in the evening I always include a fresh salad or vegetables.

Jane's story first appeared in Cambridge's newletter in 1990. Since then, Jane has managed to maintain her weight at just over 9st. "I have managed to stay at my target weight for nearly 15 years! The biggest change in me has been my self confidence and I love meeting people." Jane has remained close friends with Helen Gardiner, and still sees her every month "She continues to encourage me, and keep me on the straight and narrow. Thanks a million Cambridge!" says Jane, who won Cambridge's Long-Term maintenance Award in 2001.

# Part Three - The Cambridge Discovery

# The Perfect Food

# 10

In the United Kingdom – and elsewhere all around the world – tens of thousands now take their 'Cambridge' every day, either for weight management or as a healthy, nutritional supplement. Cambridge is a food product as acceptable as cornflakes or an apple.

For those who are overweight and following the Cambridge 'Sole Source' programme, complete nutrition is obtainable in just over 400 kcal. The major ingredients are natural and each Cambridge 'meal' consists of common foodstuffs, fortified with synthetic vitamins, minerals and trace elements. I consider that Cambridge is the perfect food for many of us, from a nutritional point of view. There is no food naturally obtainable that contains all known nutrients in so few calories.

Much of our knowledge about the importance of many nutrients in our diet arises from agricultural research. A great deal more money has been spent on the nutrition of farm animals than on that of human beings. For many years, animal feeds have been supplemented and fortified with additional vitamins and minerals. As a result, the animals are fitter and healthier, milk yields are larger and the carcases contain more protein.

My first job as a young scientist at the Dunn Nutrition Laboratory, Cambridge, was to prepare a nutritionally complete diet for guinea pigs. The diet, in fact, consisted of a mixture of clearly defined foodstuffs, such as milk protein, starch and oil, fortified with all the known vitamins and minerals. The guinea pigs thrived on it, and their growth rate was very much better than on their 'natural' diet of oats and bran. During my stay at this laboratory, tons of the new diet were used in our experiments. One day I remarked to one of my assistants, 'I wonder if we as human beings will ever eat such a terrible concoction?' He laughed and said, 'I hope not!'

My nutritional training in those early days was of enormous benefit in formulating the Cambridge Diet much later on. The guinea pig diet was always in the back of my mind. Maybe it wasn't such a terrible concoction as we thought. The guinea pigs certainly liked it. Flavoured with vanilla, strawberry or chocolate, it is possible that many people would have found it acceptable and enjoyable. Indeed it is very curious that the perfect foodstuff has never been developed before – just for nutrition.

Over the years, many dietary regimes devised by doctors have been wrtten about in books which have become best sellers. Among the most popular and successful are the Scarsdale Diet and the Atkins Diet  which are based on the principle of a low carbohydrate intake.The idea behind these diets is that consuming carbohydrate makes you hungry and by drastically reducing carbohydrate you can stick to your diet better because you are not hungry. The problem is that the above mentioned diets do not contain all the nutrients – the vitamins, minerals and trace elements – you need and in the long term will lead to serious nutritional deficiencies. This is one of the reasons leading nutritionists have advised against them.

The Cambridge Diet is low in carbohydrate and is successful for exactly the same reason: you lose your hunger. However, because it is nutritionally complete, it ensures that over the long term it will not cause the nutritional complications that you could get using a low calorie diet of food only. Cambridge have devised a programme of just under 800 kcal per day (see Chapter 2, Step 2), consisting of fish or meat and low carbohyhydrate vegetables in addition to three servings of Cambridge Diet. This programme is an excellent and more balanced substitute for the Scarsdale and Atkins diets. Moreover, it allows you the pleasure of eating and enjoying a highly palatable and healthy meal at least once a day (see also Chapter 17 - Questions and Answers).

There are a few foods on the market enriched with vitamins and minerals, but most of these have a number of defects. Usually, they do not contain *everything* necessary, and their calorie content is too high. Quite often they are meant only for sick people, and their palatability leaves much to be desired. What has happened by chance is that, though originally intended for slimming, the Cambridge Diet has become accepted by many people as a staple food in its own right. By taking the Cambridge Diet, we can receive all the benefits of complete nutrition in a very palatable form, just as farm animals have been doing for years.

Many flavours of the Cambridge Diet, available as soups and milk shakes, are made by fortifying milk and soya products. However, there is no reason why any mixture of foods could not be similarly fortified. In present day society, many people consume what nutritionists term "junk food", particularly snacks and confectionery. There is no reason why "junk food" should not be fortified to make it nutritious too.

# The Research

11

My interest in obesity began, as it has done for many others, from a personal need to lose weight. At the age of thirty I found myself fat and unhealthy. I had read books on diets and had become an 'expert' on ways to lose weight. Nothing seemed to work for me. I did find it very easy to lose about 5-10lb (2-4kg) but then quickly put the weight back on again. So I decided to accept the challenge of creating a better treatment for the overweight, using myself as a guinea pig.

My first attempt was the commercial introduction – with a local milling company – of a very high protein slimming loaf, which was made from vegetables but had the same protein content as steak – at half the price! The idea was that people could eat as much of this loaf as they liked, and eventually, because it would stem their appetite they would eat less. Altogether, with additional food, I was eating about 1,000 calories per day. In the short term it worked quite well for me and quite a few others. In a group of patients supervised by local general practitioners, patients lost about 10-15lb (4-6kg), although it took several months to achieve it.

Through the press publicity about this loaf, I achieved a certain notoriety and was often asked to speak at public and scientific meetings. While I was not exactly thrilled by the results, at least this early work was sufficient to stimulate me to further and better research.

At this time, in the early 1960s, there were very few scientists working on problems of the overweight and there was no scientific society where people interested in research could meet and discuss their results. With a group of friends, a steering committee was formed which eventually established the Association for the Study of Obesity (ASO), which still meets several times a year.

As a first step to getting the new association off the ground, I accepted the responsibility of organizing a conference on obesity in London in 1968 and delegated myself to summarize and review the latest treatments of obesity by means of diet. This involved a great deal of reading. To my amazement I found that in the past ten years many physicians had given up using food diets and had resorted to complete starvation – the Zero Calorie Diet – as the most effective way of producing weight-loss. I was not very happy with what I read. The diet could only be used by patients in hospital and then it had one very major side effect, a very serious one – death! There were at least five publications recording death in a number of patients treated by complete starvation – mostly were from cardiac problems. It was quite clear that starvation really could not be used because of the high risk. Nevertheless, I was very impressed with the magnificent weight-losses achieved. For instance, in one large trial, men lost 35lb (16kg) and women lost 26lb (11kg). Other studies showed that people could lose as much as 70lb (31.75kg) in three and a half months.

## The decision to collaborate

One of my colleagues on the Management Committee of the ASO was Dr Ian McLean Baird, of the West Middlesex Hospital, London. He acted as Chairman. He was one of the most influential and best respected physicians in the field, having already published a great deal on the health risk of obesity and on its high incidence in the British population. He also had access to hospital beds for research, and indicated that should I ever come up with a good idea he would be glad to collaborate. Like me, he saw that the combination of a nutritionist with experience in obesity research and a good all-round physician would make a strong team.

A year or so after the symposium, when we were dealing with the proceedings of the First National Meeting on Obesity, I discussed with Dr McLean Baird the subject of the Zero Calorie Diet. I had been impressed with the weight-losses and the ability of the patients to stick to what must have been a ghastly regime – water and vitamin tablets. Surely, I speculated, there must be some nutritional formulation that could be devised with fewer calories than conventional diets (which at that time were about 800 calories) and yet provide sufficient nutrients to be safe. He agreed.

And so, in 1970, Dr McLean Baird and I decided to collaborate on developing the perfect diet which we hoped would have all the desirable properties of a complete starvation regime, in that it would produce excellent weight-loss, but would also be free from side effects, and certainly would *not* result in the death of the patient.

## The Key to the Problem

The literature on the subject at that time was very sparse. Some work had been done in the 1930s on food diets of about 400 to 500 calories, but they had been virtually forgotten. No one knew if they were safe for the very long periods needed to treat severely obese patients. The key to the problem was to find out why death had occurred in patients using the complete starvation diet and then to come up with ways of preventing it. One young girl, who had been on a Zero Calorie Diet for over six months, died with damage to her heart muscle. Autopsy revealed her heart to be very thin and severely damaged, due, it was thought, to the absence of protein in the diet, so that her tissues had wasted during the course of the treatment. Thus, it was clear that the safe diet had to ensure that protein losses from the body were very small, otherwise damage could be done to the vital organs, such as heart, liver and lungs.

Protein losses can be determined by measuring nitrogen excretion in the urine and stools. If the amount of nitrogen excreted is greater than the intake, there is a 'negative nitrogen balance'. Our aim was to achieve, if possible, nitrogen equilibrium – that is, when the amount of nitrogen excreted is equal to that taken in.

The other danger in complete starvation is the excessive loss of electrolytes – such as sodium and potassium. Although most physicians using the Zero Calorie Diet added electrolytes and vitamins, this was not always done, and it was quite clear that in some cases the patient had suffered from deficiency of essential items. Any diet, to be safe, has to contain all the vitamins, minerals and trace elements.

People in conditions of complete starvation within a few days develop 'ketosis'. This is due to the incomplete combustion of fat in which certain chemicals, called ketones, accumulate in the blood and eventually spill over into the urine. In a normal diet, the presence of carbohydrate enables the fat to be broken down completely, leaving no detectable ketones in the blood and urine. Ketones have a very similar effect on the brain to alcohol. In small doses they make people feel good, happy and euphoric. In large doses, however, they can, like alcohol, have severe disadvantages, making the person feel aggressive, out of sorts and unwell. It was obvious that we had to find the critical amount of carbohydrate necessary to give a *small* level of ketones, which would be beneficial to the patient and produce a feeling of well being. Before we started, this quantity was unknown.

Carbohydrate is also important as a medium for retaining sodium and potassium in the body. Thus, inclusion of carbohydrates in the diet also stems the loss of these important electrolytes.

To summarize, we had to find the correct quantity of protein to be included in the diet, so that nitrogen losses would be as small as possible and carbohydrate had to be included to prevent excessive ketosis and to retain electrolytes.

## The Initial Plan

At first we decided to carry out some studies on patients at the West Middlesex Hospital using formula diets which would include all the known nutrients, vitamins, minerals, trace elements and essential fatty acids. We felt it was very important that the patients should be carefully monitored using a battery of clinical and laboratory examinations so as to establish if the formulas were safe or not.

Experimental trials started in June 1970. The first patients were chosen from a long waiting list. They were four women and one man, all severely overweight and all had tried relentlessly to lose weight on other diet plans but had failed to do so. Their weights ranged from 15st 7lb (220lb - 100kg) to 24st (350lb 159kg), and they were in hospital from 21 weeks up to one year.

In order to determine the smallest amount of protein and carbohydrate consistent with safety, the patients were given a variety of different formulas, starting each new one every few weeks. In addition to vitamins, minerals, trace elements and essential fatty acids a mixture of amino acids were given instead of protein. This was originally formulated for use by astronauts, and was considered to be nutritionally equivalent to a perfect protein. At first, carbohydrate was omitted and only protein given in gradually increasing quantities. Later on, small quantities of carbohydrate were added in the form of maltodextrins, a breakdown product of starch. The results were quite astonishing. Very small amounts of carbohydrate were found to have a dramatic effect on how much protein the body needed. Only about 30 grams (one ounce) of carbohydrate was enough to cut the requirement of protein by half. It was immediately apparent that the perfect diet required a finely tuned balance of carbohydrate and protein and that the total number of calories needed was smaller than ever expected – a mere 200 to 300 calories per day.

After much juggling with different formulas, we found that the minimum amounts needed were:

protein            15 grams per day and
carbohydrate       30 to 45 grams per day.

There were strong grounds for believing that diets containing such small quantities of nutrients were safe. Nitrogen losses were extremely small, as were also losses of very important minerals, such as sodium and potassium.

Our first five patients were delighted with their excellent weight-losses which averaged more than 4lb (1.8kg) a week throughout the whole study. At the end of the experiment they were in better health than when they started.

During the course of the trial we made some interesting conclusions, comparing the different dietary regimes. When receiving no calories at all, most of the patients felt very unwell, and spent most of their time in bed with headaches and muscle cramps. When they started getting a few calories they felt so much better that we could not keep them in their rooms. They became very active and spent a lot of time visiting and chatting to other patients at the hospital. So happy were they that special tasks around the hospital had to be found to keep their minds occupied.

## The Second Trial

At this stage (in the summer of 1973) everything looked extremely promising, but to ensure that the diet was safe we had to experiment on a much larger group of patients. In the next trial, we had as many as fifty patients. Our chief problem was the limited availability of hospital beds, so – to solve this problem – patients were taken into hospital for only the first three weeks and were then seen as outpatients thereafter.

While in hospital they got over their initial hunger pangs and became motivated to continue as outpatients. The safety of the diet was investigated throughout using a large number of laboratory tests, usually carried out at weekly intervals.

At this point, the diet was radically changed in protein content because the amino acid mixture proved much too expensive for use on a large scale. The new protein source chosen was an egg albumin. Many experts consider this to be the 'perfect protein', since it contains a balanced spectrum of aminoacids. In addition, the vitamins and minerals were included in the powder rather than giving them separately as a supplement.

Over the six month period, the average weight-loss was 2.5lb (1.1kg) a week. At 18 weeks, the average weight-loss was 45lb (20kg) – not bad, considering we were dealing with outpatients. The weight loss was, of course, not as great as we had seen in hospitalized patients. Quite a few of the outpatients dropped out and others found it very difficult to remain faithful to the programme. This was entirely understandable. The patients cheated because the mixture had a very unpleasant taste and it was more like taking a dose of medicine than food. There was no doubt in my mind that this concoction was much too unpalatable to present to the general public: people might try it for a short time but eventually they would give up. Nevertheless, these second trials (which lasted three years) were a huge success. None of the patients developed any significant abnormality while on the diet. They felt and looked well. We were convinced that we were on the right track.

## A Question of Hunger

The major question was whether overweight people would ever be able to follow the course as outpatients without the initial hospitalization. We knew that it took a few days to get over the early hunger pangs and this might be too much for most people to tolerate. They would eventually cheat and not stick to the diet.

At this time (early 1975) a new appetite suppressant drug, Mazindol, had been released on to the market. It was claimed to be the most highly effective drug of its kind ever developed, without any side effects. The combination of this drug and our diet seemed ideal. We designed a study in which twenty patients took the new appetite suppressant while twenty others were given dummy tablets. Each group took its tablets for four weeks and then they changed over and took the other one instead. Quite early on in the trial it became clear which patients were taking the drug, because of the side effects many of them suffered, such as nausea, sleep loss, palpitations and high euphoria. In some cases we had to stop the tablets altogether since the drug was so badly tolerated. It began to look as though the experiment would turn out to be a complete disaster. On analyzing the results, however, we were quite amazed.

Those taking the appetite suppressant received no special benefits, and virtually everybody who consumed the diet, whatever the tablet they were given, lost weight. This was good news, as it showed that people could get over the initial feeling of hunger without the additional need of an appetite suppressant, with all the nasty side effects. We found we could allow our patients to use the diet at home on an outpatient basis, rather than their being admitted to hospital.

Although we knew that in hospital the patients were not hungry when consuming the diet, it seemed incredible that the same could happen to outpatients. We had created the same lack of hunger which occurs in complete starvation, yet the patients were able to live normal lives without the constraints of hospital. Our eight week study showed again that the regime was perfectly safe from the clinical viewpoint.

This breakthrough was what we had been looking for and provided the opportunity to carry out large numbers of studies on very many patients, not only in London but in Cambridge and elsewhere. Shortly afterwards, Professor Ivor Mills, Head of the Department of Medicine in Cambridge, agreed to set up the obesity clinic at Addenbrooke's Hospital at which I and one of his senior registrars saw thirty patients each week. This speeded up the development of the diet enormously.

## The Cambridge Diet Appears

Before we started the next study we considered the protein source. We had found that there were several disadvantages in using egg albumin, even though it had high nutritional value. It was poor in taste and it would coagulate in hot drinks. It also proved to be expensive. In the spring of 1976 we turned instead to skimmed milk, which is an excellent source of casein and other milk proteins, and consulted with food technologists to work on the flavourings. Eventually, after a great deal of work, a 'not too unpalatable' complete diet was achieved. It contained 330 calories comprising 33 grams of protein, 44 grams of carbohydrate and 3 grams of fat. The flavours were chicken and asparagus soups and banana, peach, raspberry and strawberry drinks. This was to become the basis of the Cambridge Diet, which we hoped would be available eventually to millions of people.

It was important to examine the results of the next experiment carefully. We needed to check that the new formulation was safe, and this could only be done at the Metabolic Ward at the West Middlesex Hospital. Yet the ultimate use of the formulation was to be by outpatients. The obvious answer was a study in which we compared outpatients and inpatients. Altogether, a total of fifty obese patients were given the new flavoured formulation for between 4-12 weeks. After four weeks the mean weight-loss was 20lb (9kg) in hospitalized patients and 16lb (7.25kg) in outpatients. After eight weeks, both groups had lost a mean of 24lb (11kg). At first these results sound surprising. What had happened was that at the sixth week the hospitalized patients had been discharged and allowed to go home on an 800 calorie diet. The final weights of the two groups indicated that there was no great advantage in taking people into hospital, with all the trouble and expense that entailed. The weight-losses as outpatients could be equally good.

This was a very important trial, the summation of all the work done over an eight-year period. As in other trials, the question of safety was all-important. Nitrogen balance was studied and it was shown that nitrogen losses were very small. Serum electrolytes were examined. Monthly electrocardiographs indicated no changes. The tests were remarkable in showing that the patients who used the diet were fit and well.

Our findings, to which A Grant, O Edwards and ER Littlewood also lent their names, were published in a refereed report in the December issue of *The International Journal of Obesity* in 1978. It was this paper which led directly to the launching of the Cambridge Diet in the United States in 1980, because it was read by Jack Feather, a wealthy Californian, who decided it was worth doing something positive about it. The story is told in Chapter 13.

# The Clinics

## 12

## In Practice

Much of the work towards the end of the research period was carried out at Addenbrooke's Hospital in Cambridge, where an Obesity Clinic was specially set up for work on the Cambridge Diet. Within a few weeks, there were some 40 obese patients who came for treatment regularly.

The treatment of obesity was not a popular subject among hospital doctors. Before the advent of the Cambridge Diet, overweight patients usually attended regular clinics and were then referred to the hospital dietician, who, more often than not, recommended a conventional 800-1000 calorie diet. They rarely lost weight and doctors were not specifically involved. However, with the new treatment, using the Cambridge Diet, an Obesity Clinic became very rewarding. Obese patients can be the most interesting of characters and it was extremely satisfying to see them succeeding for the first time in their lives, and to join in the enthusiasm their success created. The doctors often remarked that it was the most enjoyable clinic they held.

## The Enthusiastic Physicians

We were joined by a number of other groups in Europe and in the United States, and from all these clinics came enthusiastic reports that the weight-losses were excellent and that the Diet appeared to be very safe.

Dr JH Paul Wilson of Rotterdam, for example, thought the new formula was a major advance in therapy for the massively obese patients who, on conventional diets, would need many years to achieve their ideal weight. Using the new formula he found that patients could lose between 3-4½lb (1.3 – 2kg) a week consistently. Of the 90 patients he studied, a substantial number stayed on the diet for three or four months and some for as long as 11 months. They had an average weight-loss of 22lb (10kg) in four weeks and no serious side effects were seen. One woman started at 24st 12lb (348lb - 158kg) – and lost 187lb (85kg)  in 15 months, achieving her ideal weight of 10st 10lb (150lb - 68kg) – which he considered a remarkable achievement in view of previous failure on other diets.

Dr Noel Hickey, of Dublin, reported that on the basis of his own clinical trials the VLCD was a remarkable advance in medical treatment and quite different from 'crash diets' extremely popular among the public. He found the new formula was extremely successful in producing very substantial weight reduction of the same order as that seen in complete starvation, without all the associated hazards.

In Ireland, and elsewhere, most doctors are reluctant to put patients on conventional diets, because the dropout rate is so high and people regain all the weight lost within a year or two. It is here that the new formulation scores: because patients lose a great deal of weight rapidly, they are stimulated to change their eating habits so as to achieve permanent weight-loss.

At his clinic, he studied 14 people in which the average weight-losses at four weeks were 17lb (7kg) for men and 11½lb (5kg) for women. At eight weeks the mean weight-losses were 29lb (13kg) for men and 18½lb (8kg) for women. Such results are impossible to achieve using conventional diets. Although they were consuming only 330 calories, the patients lost their hunger after only a few days on the diet, a fact which I found very impressive.

## The Critics

Not everyone in the scientific community approved of the Cambridge Diet. After its launch in the USA, and later in the UK, there was a flood of articles, notes and reviews criticizing the Cambridge Diet. Among the most vociferous was the leader writer of the Journal of the American Medical Association, who claimed the diet was dangerous and – in support of this claim – drew attention to the small loss of lean body mass which occurs while on the diet. What the JAMA failed to appreciate was that any overweight individual would lose lean body mass on **any** weight-loss programme.

Lean body mass is defined as 'the total weight of the body minus its fatty tissue'. For instance, if you weigh just over 14st (200lb - 91kg) and have 80lb (36kg) of fatty tissue, your lean body mass is 120lb (55kg). Basically it consists of the skeleton and the soft tissues of the body, particularly the muscles.

Using some very sophisticated measuring techniques, Dr Phillip James in the UK showed that overweight people had much more lean body mass than their lean counterparts. This is a logical finding, because if an individual has a lot of body fat to carry around, he will need a lot of muscle to support it. To give an example, if a man is 50lb (23kg) overweight, about 36 per cent or 18lb (8kg) of this excess weight is lean body mass. This is equivalent to about 4lb (2kg) of protein, a quantity much larger than anyone ever anticipated and which provides a substantial store of this nutrient. If the 50lb (23kg) over weight man goes on a diet and reaches his ideal weight, his body will receive an extra bonus of 4lb (2kg) of protein to use for his nutritional needs. This loss of protein and lean body mass occurs on **any** diet whenever weight is lost, not just the Cambridge Diet.

In our original work on the development of the Cambridge Diet, we carefully measured the nitrogen losses occurring in patients while in hospital. It was found that over a four-week period, the difference between nitrogen intake and that excreted was only 55 grams. This is equivalent to about 0.75lb protein. From the weight-loss which had occurred could be calculated the amount of nitrogen excreted due to the loss of body protein, which must of necessity arise during weight-loss. It was established that the nitrogen excreted was no greater than one would expect in a person losing that particular amount of weight.

One of the charges made by the JAMA experts was that if loss of lean body mass does occur it could come from the heart. Again, their criticism might apply to any weight-loss diet. There is absolutely no evidence that there are changes to the heart muscle in patients using the Cambridge Diet. Studies have been conducted on hundreds of patients in metabolic wards and in outpatients clinics, in many centres in Europe and the United States and *no* heart changes associated with the Cambridge Diet have been seen. This even applies when studies were continued on patients using the Diet for up to four months as sole source. One of the techniques used by the cardiologists at three different centres was continuous twenty-four hour monitoring of heart rhythms using a tape recorder. No changes were seen in any significance while patients were on the Cambridge Diet.

None of the scientists who criticized the diet had ever used it in their clinics, whereas the reality – in both the USA and the UK – speaks very much against their conclusions. Many general practitioners, after a few months, found that the Cambridge Diet was effective and very safe. They realized that with their limited time it was impossible to treat all the overweight patients in their practice individually. So they would hand them over to the nurse (who really didn't have any time for the patient, either). The solution was to bring in a well trained Cambridge Counsellor. Of course, if the patient was extremely overweight and wanted to use the 'Sole Source' programme for periods of several months, then the doctor would see that person regularly, but otherwise he would not need to spend his valuable time in this manner.

## Other Beneficial Effects

Many of the doctors who studied the Cambridge Diet were specialists in a wide number of medical subjects, such as nutrition, endocrinology, diabetes and cardiovascular disease. Besides weight-loss, they were also interested in the subsidiary beneficial effects of the Diet, several of which came to light. Much of this was reported at two scientific conferences on the Cambridge Diet, in October 1980 and June 1983.

## Diabetes

The risk of developing diabetes is very high in overweight people. In fact, the majority of adults who become diabetic are overweight, and most doctors, on examining a diabetic for the first time, will recommend weight-loss as an important part of their treatment. Diabetics, like most other overweight people, find it extremely difficult to lose weight and maintain their weight-loss on conventional diets. With an introduction of the Cambridge Diet their lives have been made much easier, because they can also succeed.

One doctor, with a particular interest in diabetes, put a number of overweight mild diabetics on the Cambridge Diet as their sole form of treatment for six weeks. After a few days, their blood sugar became normal and their high blood fats (cholesterol and triglycerides) also decreased. These beneficial changes continued until the end of their treatment. Other doctors have found that, when treating diabetics with the Cambridge Diet, it is necessary to reduce patients' medication..

## Blood Fats

The treatment of high blood fats had been of special interest to me and Dr Ian McLean Baird for many years. It was therefore very encouraging for us to find that the Cambridge Diet reduced blood cholesterol by 25 per cent and triglycerides by 40 per cent. Every single patient who follows the Cambridge 'Sole Source' weight-loss programme shows a decrease in blood fat, especially those who had high levels to start with. Most of these people, who were at high risk for coronary heart disease, were able to get their blood fats down to normal by using the diet. However, this was only achieved while they were using 'Sole Source'. On returning to a normal diet their blood fats increased again, although not to such high levels as were seen previously.

## High Blood Pressure

It is very common for the overweight person to suffer from high blood pressure. A drop in blood pressure is seen within a few days of starting the diet, even when weight-loss is still quite small. On achievement of normal weight, blood pressure is often brought down completely to normal. To give an example, one patient, Robert Walton of Little Paxton reported the following:

'My wife works for a doctor, and one day he asked several of us if he could try out his new blood pressure machine, using us as patients. I was most happy to oblige as I was quite sure I had no problems with my blood pressure. You can imagine my surprise, and the doctor's concern, when my blood pressure registered 200/130! As I am only 36 years of age, it didn't seem possible. In fact, he even took it again, and when it remained the same we all thought there might be something wrong with the machine. As it turned out, the machine was correct.

'At about this time [early May 1984] friends introduced me to the Cambridge Diet. My weight was 14st 3lb (199lb - 90kg). I went on the diet as my sole source of nutrition for one month and by 30th May my blood pressure registered 150/105! I had a one-week maintenance period and then went back sole source for another week. By 6th June my blood pressure was 145/ 93 and kept going down until 29th June when it reached 125/90. 1 had lost the weight I had been trying to get off and then weighed 12st 10lb (169lb - 76kg), a loss of 30lb (13kg).

'By taking the Cambridge Diet for weight maintenance and for nutrition, I have easily been able to keep my blood pressure at a normal range. The doctor has been quite amazed at my progress and fully encourages me to stay with the Cambridge Diet formula as a means of controlling my blood pressure.'

The standard treatment of high blood pressure is to give medication. Unfortunately, the drugs do not cure the condition and therefore have to be taken for very long periods, often for life. Throughout the world there are millions of people affected and the total cost of medication is enormous. If weight reduction, using the Cambridge Diet, could cause a permanent decrease in blood pressure in even a proportion of those affected, there would be a great saving in both time and money.

## Anti-depressants

One of the problems of slimming diets is that patients often become depressed. This has not been a complication of the Cambridge Diet; in fact, the reverse is true and people often report that they have never felt happier in the whole of their lives. Dr Russell Cook of Addenbrooke's Hospital, had a special interest in depression and decided to investigate this aspect using some sophisticated questionnaires which he had devised.

For his study, he used the antidepressant drug, Miaserin. Half the patients were treated with the drug and the remainder with a dummy tablet. Altogether thirty patients were given the Cambridge Diet sole source for sixteen weeks. He found that most patients on the Cambridge Diet were not depressed at all and that Miaserin made no difference to their state of mind, or weight-loss. Although the study was negative from his point of view, in that the drug had no beneficial effect, the information he obtained coincidentally about the diet was most helpful. From a variety of biochemical and clinical tests, he found that the thirty patients were healthy and well at the end of the sixteen weeks. It was his work that gave us great confidence to treat large number of patients at the obesity clinic for long periods of time, often six to nine months, knowing that the treatment was safe. In fact, it is as safe from six to nine months as it is at four to eight weeks.

## Future Research in Obesity

When this book was first written – in 1985 – much more research into the cause of obesity was needed. Of course, everyone knows that people become overweight because they consume more energy (calories) than they expend. On the other hand, there are thin people with very healthy appetites who consume large amounts of food without getting fat. That research has continued and – as the worldwide concern over obesity and overweight increases – will continue for the foreseeable future.

In 1986, a book for professionals about the Cambridge diet was written by myself and Dr John Marks. This book (recently revised and obtainable from the Cambridge Manufacturing Company on request)details all of the research on VLCDs which has taken place in the past and more recently. It is recommended reading for those professionals who are interested in learning more on the subject. For the Cambridge organisation there are a number of landmark events:

☐ In 1987, the UK Department of Health – through their COMA committee published a report on VLCDs in which a panel of experts examined their use and satèty. They concluded that VLCDs – especially the Cambridge Diet were safe when used correctly and made a small number of recommendations. In summary, they said that they could be used with safety for up to tour weeks in healthy individuals and that after that people should be under medical supervision. Those with medical problems should consult their doctor before use and COMA listed a number of contraindications. They recommended a small increase in the protein content of the original diet and said that men should take four packets a day instead of three. All their recommendations were adopted by Cambridge, although this involved considerable expense in changing packaging and printing. We were extremely satisfied when the COMA committee clearly approved of the use of the Cambridge Diet with modifications.

☐ Early in the 1990s, the American Medical Association and the American Dietetic Association highly recommended VLCDs for the treatment of obesity – especially under medical supervision. Thus the American establishment – which had been so critical of VLCDs when they first came out – changed their minds when they saw how valuable and safe they were in practice.

☐ In 1993, 'The Swansea Trial' edited by Dr Steve Kreitzman and myself was published to counter the continuing controversy over the loss of protein tissue. It contained clinical research – conducted by three universities ( Swansea ,Leeds, and Cambridge) and Howard Foundation Research – which clearly settled the controversy over the loss of protein during weight reduction – 'the results showed that the loss of protein with the Cambridge Diet, is no greater than would he expected on any diet during weight reduction'. This view has now been finally accepted by the scientific community (for further and later information consult FES website: www.foodedsoc.org.)

Research on VLCDs has continued and a number of important papers are worth summarising:

♦ Our 8-year experience strongly suggests that the I VLCD approach using high quality protein supplement and multi-disciplinary counselling provides a reasonable success rate for achieving and maintaining weight loss in the morbidity obese population. (Kirschner et al, 1988)

♦ The short-term use of a VLCD is very effective in rapidly improving glycaemic control and promoting substantial weight loss in obese patients with Type 2 diabetes. Moreover, a VLCD increases insulin secretion and reduces substrate for gluconeogenesis. Thus VLCD treatment may improve glycaemic control by factors more than caloric restriction alone. (Capstick et al, 1997)

♦ A VLCD program is suitable for preoperative weight reduction in morbid obesity and seems not to compromise the immune system. (Pekkarinen &Mustajoki, 1997)

♦ Substantial weight loss and improvement in cardiovascular risk factors could be maintained for 1 year in Type 2 diabetic patients by the use of a very low calorie diet. (Paisley et al, 1998)

♦ VLEDs are a proven success in achieving significant short-term reduction in body weight. There is evidence to suggest that meal replacements may make a contribution to the maintenance of weight loss in some individuals. (Jebb & Goldberg, 1998)

♦ This weight loss programme with a VLCD enabled obese subjects to lose weight and decrease cardiovascular risks. Despite some regain in weight during follow-up, the beneficial effects were overall maintained over the year. (Pekkarinen et al, 1998)

♦ This four-compartment analysis of changes in body composition provides no evidence of any significant loss of protein in this treatment programme. However if two-compartment models are used to assess changes in body composition during acute weight loss the very significant loss of water will appear as losses of lean tissue. (Jebb et al, 1998)

♦ VLCD was most efficacious if combined with behaviour modification and active follow-up. The literature on long-term follow-up of dietary treatment of obesity points to an overall median success rate of 15% and a possible adjuvant effect of group therapy, behaviour modification and active follow-up. (Ayyad & Andersen, 2000)

♦ Greater initial weight loss as the first step of weight management may result in improved weight maintenance. (Astrup & Rossner, 2000)

♦ VLEDs accomplish maximum initial loss and can be conducted safely in patients with obesity associated diseases – diabetes, hypertension, or other chronic diseases. (Astrup & Rossner, 2000)

♦ VLCD with active follow-up treatment seems to be one of the better treatment modalities related to long term weight maintenance success. (Saris, 2001)

♦ Five years after completing structured weight-loss programme, the average individual maintained a weight loss of >3kg and a reduced weight of >3% of initial body weight. After VLEDs, or weight loss of >20kg, individuals maintained significantly more weight loss than after HBDs* or weight losses of <10kg. (Anderson et al, 2001)

* HBD = hypoenergetic balanced diet is a diet of around 1200-1500kcal consisting of conventional food

# The Road to Success

*13*

## Finding the Funds

Research is expensive. It requires facilities, salaried technical staff and money to pay for chemicals and routine analyses. Before embarking on new projects, every scientist has to ensure that suitable funds are available. In 1970, when work on the diet started, research support from government sources, such as the Medical Research Council, was severely curtailed. Those of us engaged in the research relied chiefly on pharmaceutical companies, which were often willing to invest in a project which might be of commercial interest to them.

In January 1970, the medical weekly, the *Lancet,* carried an advertisement from a company named Vivonex, asking if anyone was interested in research on their product. On further inquiry, I discovered that Vivonex was a complete diet of 2,000 calories, which had been developed for astronauts undertaking space missions. The idea was to produce a completely synthetic food substitute, composed of a mixture of aminoacids, which left little or no residue, so that stools from astronauts could be kept to a minimum. Unfortunately, astronauts preferred real food and were not satisfied with the unpalatable mixture Vivonex had prepared. Nevertheless, I saw that it might be possible to modify the Vivonex formula into the perfect slimming diet. I contacted the company in California and they agreed, through their London representative, to supply research funds. Materials were flown over from Mountain View, California, to London so that the work could begin.

The project had been under way for only a few months, when we learned that the Vivonex Corporation had been taken over by Morton Norwich, a large American company, but the new owners acknowledged that our work was important and interesting, and agreed to continue supporting it.

By the end of 1971, the first trial with the Vivonex mixture was completed, and the results were astonishing. It was possible, it seemed, for fat people to live on as little as 250 calories per day. My patent agent assured me that the diet was an original concept and I decided to register a provisional patent application in the United Kingdom in March 1972.

The next twelve months saw very active discussions with Morton Norwich, to ascertain their interest and, as a result, a satisfactory license agreement was worked out. One year later, patent applications were applied for in twelve other countries, including the United States. Morton Norwich decided to meet the patent costs and to provide finance for staff salaries and all outgoing expenses. To clinch the deal, I flew out to Norwich, New York, calling at Philadelphia on the way to pick up my United States lawyer and patent agent. The latter turned out to be an amateur pilot and I still have sleepless nights remembering that single-engine plane trip from Philadelphia to Norwich, New York!

Everything went well for a time – the egg albumin diet had been successful – and then to our dismay, Morton Norwich replaced their President with someone who did not look favourably on our research, and our project was dropped, which seemed catastrophic as I now had to look for somebody else to support the work.

My attempts to secure new funding were disappointing until the intervention of Dennis Jones. Dennis was an old student of mine who later joined the large multinational company, Organon. Through his introduction, I became an adviser to Organon and later I put the idea to Dennis that Organon might be interested in supporting our pioneer work on dieting. He eventually convinced Organon of the worthiness of the project, and we enjoyed a very happy collaboration with Organon, with Dennis as the project leader.

## The Howard Diet

The first step in making the new diet was to find a factory capable of manufacturing the basic diet material to my specifications. The company chosen belonged to Lyons Tetley at Market Harborough, about 50 miles from Cambridge, where technical staff had become experts in devising soups and milk shakes. My formula – which now used skimmed milk as a protein source – was converted into chicken and asparagus soups, as well as banana, raspberry, peach and strawberry milk shakes. These flavours were a great improvement on what had been developed before and received a tolerant, if unenthusiastic, response from patients.

The so-called 'Howard Diet' was then tested in a number of centres, principally Addenbrooke's Hospital in Cambridge and the West Middlesex Hospital in lsleworth, just as if it had been a new drug. Each patient was seen weekly, and frequent samples of blood were taken for biochemical analysis. After a study of several hundred patients, using a battery of routine tests, including electrocardiographs and other clinical examinations, the diet was found remarkably effective, and absolutely no adverse effects of any importance were discovered.

Yet Organon did not wish to rely solely on the results from the two obesity clinics, and enrolled six other clinics in different parts of Europe to evaluate the Howard Diet. Organon had good contacts with Dr Paul Wilson and Dr Steven Lamberts at the Department of Internal Medicine at the University of Rotterdam, and also with Dr Noel Hickey, Dr Geoffrey Bourke and Dr Risteard Mulcahy at University Hospital, Dublin. At this time, I was already giving lectures throughout Europe on the new diet and had been particularly well received in Copenhagen, Gothenburg and Naples. All these groups decided to take part in formal trials. In addition, Dr Harold Shapiro in Manchester, a general practitioner with a large obesity practice, decided to compare the Howard Diet with his standard 600 calorie food diet. Altogether, eight centres were involved in the final testing. Without exception they agreed that the diet was extremely effective and quite safe.

Randolph de Bruin, head of the Clinical Department at Organon, produced an enthusiastic report. He had been especially interested in the trials at Rotterdam, because of his personal associations with Dr Paul Wilson. However, not everyone supported it. Organon had also conducted palatability trials in France and reported that the general acceptance of the taste was not encouraging and that he was sceptical whether ordinary members of the public would take to the diet. He was no doubt right to pronounce the diet poor in taste; nevertheless the dropout rate in all the trials had been extremely low, much lower than with ordinary diets. We countered his argument with our view that people on slimming diets seldom expect to be treated with the flavour of gourmet food. For six months there was silence while the Organon Board deliberated.

## Competitors

About the same time as our collaboration with Morton Norwich, two American scientists had also hit on the idea of developing a new, very low calorie treatment for massively obese diabetics. They were Saul Genuth and Victor Vertes of Cleveland, Ohio. Both our groups met at the First International Congress on Obesity in London in 1973 to present our results to the world for the first time.

(Genuth and Vertes were being supported by the Delmark Company – part of the Swiss giant pharmaceutical company, Sandoz – and their formulation, which was based on egg albumin as the source of protein, was eventually sold in the USA as Optifast and in Europe as Modifast.)

Genuth and Vertes insisted that the diet should only be used by skilled physicians who specialized in the treatment of the overweight in special clinics. Altogether they liaised with doctors on the treatment of hundreds of patients throughout the US. Their trials were very successful and like ourselves, they saw few side effects. While all this was happening in the USA, Sandoz had its eyes on Europe, particularly Germany, and they decided to speed up their marketing plans in Europe, so that Modifast was introduced to pharmacies in Germany and Holland in 1978.

Organon were well and truly beaten to the post. I believe that the Howard Diet was more palatable than Modifast. It was certainly cheaper and if it could have been launched it would have competed well.

Following the moderate commercial success of Modifast on the continent, the product was introduced into the UK in 1980, where it became available from pharmacies with the recommendation of general practitioners, who had been circularized with a great deal of literature about it.

Another country in which there was activity was Denmark. In 1978, I visited the University of Copenhagen to give a lecture at the Hvidovre Hospital to Professor Quaade and his group. He was the most respected expert in the treatment of obesity in Denmark and his prime interest at that time was in surgical operations. Together with a colleague he had developed an improved method for stomach stapling.

After my lecture on the Howard Diet, he was extremely impressed with the results obtained and felt that there might now be no need for these operations. He therefore decided to carry out a comparative study, using the Howard Diet on one or two of his patients. Although he was impressed with their weight-loss, which was equivalent to that obtained with his operations, he did not like the flavours and subsequently decided to devise his own formulation based on orange juice and soya protein. Since he was a little uncertain of the exact formulation, he asked my advice. I flew to Copenhagen and met him and his colleague, Oluf Mork, and was delighted when they agreed to formulate a new diet of almost exactly the same composition as the Howard Diet, because it would independently confirm my results. An endorsement of the safety of my diet was of greater value than any commercial considerations. Their clinical trials were very successful and Professor Quaade was able to confirm the safety of the Howard Diet in his own clinic. Oluf Mork went on to market his own 'Nupo' brand which was available in health food stores and supermarkets.

Because of its greater palatability and more effective method of distribution, it was decided to introduce the Cambridge Diet in Denmark in the spring of 1985 under the name Cambridge Kuren

## The Feathers

After many months of waiting, Organon told me that they had reluctantly decided not to proceed with the marketing of the Howard Diet. Clearly the appearance of Modifast in Germany and The Netherlands was the deciding factor and Organon accepted defeat. They wanted me to assign the patent rights to Sandoz for whatever sum Organon could get, but this was entirely unacceptable. Having spent years developing the diet, the last thing I wished to see was all the work dissipated for the sake of a rival product. Organon wanted to recoup some of their large investment, but eventually they gave up any claim they had to the patent rights, and once again I had to find another sponsor.

It was not too long before further support was found. In the summer of 1979, Jack and Eileen Feather, two Californian multimillionaires, decided to put a considerable part of their fortune into a new venture. They chose to support the Howard Diet (which then became known as the Cambridge Diet).

Jack had always been interested in nutritional research, partly because of his own experience of combatting polio as a student through a combination of nutrition and exercise. In 1975, he set about producing a new and revolutionary slimming diet. After three and a half years of work, he and his son, Vaughn, had been able to develop a product which they felt ready to market. Before doing so, the Feathers decided to take a short vacation to their summer home in England. Jack took with him on the plane a stack of scientific journals to read, including some back issues of the *International Journal of Obesity*. By the time dinner was being served, Jack had reached the 1978 December issue of the journal and our article about the Howard Diet.

Jack was quite amazed by what he read, because it was very close to the ideas which he and his son had worked on, but better. Their English home was quite close to the West Middlesex Hospital, and in no time at all they contacted Dr Ian McLean Baird and arranged a meeting. When they heard that the product was covered by a United States patent they were extremely excited and anxious to obtain the rights.

An agreement was quickly reached and the Feathers began their marketing of our diet in March of the following year. It was they who chose to change the name of the 'Howard Diet' to the Cambridge Diet, and their new company was called Cambridge Plan International.

In 1981, the Feathers introduced the system of marketing by Cambridge Counsellors, which was so much more beneficial than selling cans of diet through chemists. In their own development they had achieved considerable expertise in flavouring. The new Cambridge Diet was a huge leap ahead in palatability compared with the old Howard Diet. Overweight Americans liked the flavours and the diet became extremely successful.

## Imitators

The success of the Cambridge Diet can be measured by the number of companies which attempted to rival the formulation. Altogether, there were more than fifty. Their products were sold under the name 'Oxford Diet', 'Eton Diet', 'University Diet', and many other names, and were chiefly retailed from chemists' shops. Patent infringement actions were vigorously pursued in the courts. In South Africa, a Johannesburg entrepreneur cheekily introduced his 'NEW' Cambridge Diet, while in the United Kingdom, Univite 330, a close copy of the Cambridge Diet, was made available in 1983 by mail order and later through the counsellor-type system as 'The Micro Diet'. None of these is exactly formulated according to the results of stringent tests which produced the original 'Cambridge Diet'.

In retrospect, the decisions of Morton Norwich and Organon to drop the diet were blessings in disguise. The Feather family, in deciding to take up the Cambridge Diet made a significant contribution to medical science and the treatment of obesity in particular.

# The Story Today

## 14

My involvement with Cambridge Plan International was very limited. Although I was occasionally invited to give a lecture or was asked for advice on medical and scientific matters, the business organization was completely outside my sphere of influence.

But in Britain the situation was different. I had wanted the Diet to be available in Britain for many years but – for one reason or another – the plans had been continually postponed.

## Cambridge Nutrition

In April 1984, a decision was taken to start a new company in Britain called Cambridge Nutrition Limited, completely independent of the Feather family, headed by my brother, Dr Roger Howard, a biochemist who returned from the United States to take on the challenge of making the Diet available to the many millions of obesity sufferers in this country.

Now – in 2004 – the Cambridge Diet is produced and distributed by Cambridge Manufacturing Company Limited (CMC), which is part of the Howard Foundation Group. CMC has three divisions:

Cambridge Manufacturing

Cambridge Health and Weight Plan

Cambridge Export

*Cambridge Manufacturing* is responsible for the production and distribution of the whole range of Cambridge products for both UK and overseas customers. *Cambridge Health and Weight Plan* is responsible for marketing and it also recruits and trains the independent Cambridge Counsellors for product distribution in the UK. The division looks after media relations and produces a wide range of literature. *Cambridge Export* is responsible for overseas distributors. It seeks out potential distributors and handles contract details. It is also responsible for maintaining liaison with these independent overseas companies.

## The Howard Foundation

CMC is wholly owned by The Howard Foundation, a charitable trust established in 1982. The aims of the Foundation are to provide funding for biomedical research in the fields of obesity, nutrition and key areas of health. Further aims include the funding, the construction and maintenance of buildings at Downing

College, Cambridge University, and the establishment of scholarships for international students.

## Achievements

Donations to Downing College, Cambridge to fund construction of The Howard Building, a conference hall, completed in 1987. Later support led to Howard Court, student accommodation, completed in 1994. Several international scientific meetings have been held at Downing College with the support and sponsorship of the Foundation.

Howard Foundation Research (HFR) was established in 1986 to carry out scientific research into low calorie diets. HFR has published numerous scientific papers, most notably "The Swansea Trial" edited by Dr S N Kreitzman and Dr A Howard.

Based at Papworth Hospital, near Cambridge, the COAG Trace Elements Laboratory ran from 1991 to 2000 carrying out research into aspects of nutrition and health, especially the prevention of coronary heart disease. The equipment has since been transferred to the University of Ulster and the University Hospital in Poznan, Poland, for the continuation of research programmes.

The Howard Foundation Chair in Human Nutrition was established at the University of Ulster in 1993.

Additional research has been supported at University of Cambridge, University of Wales, Institute of Science and Technology, Imperial College of Science and Technology, Charing Cross Hospital, Guys Hospital, St George's Hospital, London, Hope Hospital, Salford (now Salford Royal) and the Universities of Swansea, Leeds and Liverpool. Outside the UK, grants have been given to the University of London, Ontario; the University of New York, NY; and Florida International University, Miami.

International meetings on low calorie diets have been supported in Israel 1986, Cambridge 1989 and Japan 1990.

## The Wider World

As we have already seen, Cambridge is available around the world, and this expansion process started in 1985, with the launch of Cambridge Kuren in Denmark. Further new markets were established in other parts of Western Europe, such as Germany and France, and then in Sweden and Norway. Cambridge is also available in Europe in The Netherlands and Belgium, Austria, Switzerland and Malta.

In 1990, Cambridge was first made available in eastern Europe, where Cambridge Dieta was launched in Poland. Further developments have taken place in the Czech Republic and negotiations are in progress in Russia.

In 1995, Cambridge was first introduced into Asia, where it is now available in Singapore, Malaysia, Thailand, The Philippines and Hong Kong. In the Middle East, distributors have been appointed in Oman and Lebanon.

A full list of distributor details is included in Appendix 3.

# Part Four – Further Useful Information

# Nutritional Information

**15**

## A Complete Diet

A complete diet by definition contains every substance the body needs for perfect health. Today, nutritionists have a wide knowledge of the role of nutrients in health and disease. We know that people need many different nutrients if they are to maintain health and reduce the risk of diet-related diseases. The amount of each nutrient needed is called the nutritional requirement. These vary for different nutrients between individuals.

Each nutrient has particular functions in the body and some nutrients are needed in larger quantities than others. For example protein is needed in gram (g) quantities. Vitamin C is needed in milligram (mg) quantities, and vitamin B12 is needed in microgram (μg or mcg) quantities. Individual requirements of each nutrient are related to a person's age, sex, level of physical activity and state of health.

## Nutritional Measures

In the UK, estimated requirements for particular groups of the population are based on advice given by the 1991 Committee on Medical Aspects of Food and Nutrition Policy (COMA). In their report, COMA defined a number of important terms:

☐ **Dietary Reference Values** (DRVs) for food energy and nutrients, which are estimates of the average requirements for groups of people and are not individual recommendations or goals. DRVs are specific to groups, such as babies, or the elderly.

☐ The **Estimated Average Requirement** (EAR) is an estimate of the average requirement for energy or a nutrient – approximately 50% of a group of people will require less, and 50% will require more. EAR is always the figure used for energy.

☐ The **Reference Nutrient Intake** (RNI) is the amount of a nutrient that is enough to ensure that the needs of nearly all the group (97.5%) are being met.

☐ The **Lower Reference Nutrient Intake** (LRNI) is the lowest of requirements for a nutrient, and only 2.5% of the population are expected to have requirements this low.

☐ In addition to these, two other measures have come into daily use: the Recommended Daily Allowance (RDA) and the Guideline Daily Amounts (GDA).

## Recommended Daily Allowance (RDA)

The term with which you will be most familiar is the Recommended Daily Allowance (RDA), which is used for food labelling. The European labelling RDA provides details for a wide range of vitamins and minerals.

## Guideline Daily Amounts

To assist UK consumers put nutrition labelling into context, Guideline Daily Amounts (GDAs) were devised for fat and energy. For example, current GDAs for energy are 2000 kcal for females and 2500 kcal for males. The GDA for fat is 70g and 95g for females and males respectively.

The Estimated Average Requirements (EAR) for energy is shown in the table below and are rounded up to give the GDA figures given above. Note that these requirements do change with age and activity levels.

| Estimated Average Requirements for energy | | |
| --- | --- | --- |
| Age | Males | Females |
| 15-18 yr | 2755 | 2110 |
| 19-50 yr | 2550 | 1940 |
| 51-59 yr | 2550 | 1900 |
| 60-64 yr | 2380 | 1900 |
| 65-74 yr | 2330 | 1900 |
| 74+ yr | 2100 | 1810 |

In comparison to adolescents, energy requirements are lower for both men and women as are requirements for calcium and phosphorus. There is also a reduced requirement in women for magnesium, and in men for iron. The requirements for protein and most of the vitamins and minerals remain virtually unchanged.

After the age of 50 in women and age 60 in men, the daily energy requirements decrease gradually. Protein requirements also decrease for men but continue to increase slightly for women. The requirements for vitamins and minerals remain virtually unchanged for both men and women. There is one exception – after the menopause, women's requirement for iron is reduced to the same level as that for men.

## Energy mix

Fat, protein and carbohydrate all provide energy, but we need to have them in the right proportions. Evidence suggests that a poor energy mix is a risk factor in various diseases such as coronary heart disease and certain cancers. The 1991 COMA panel recommended the energy mix as shown in the table, below.

| Recommended Daily Mix (%) | | |
|---|---|---|
| | (inc alcohol) | no alcohol |
| Protein | 15 | 15 |
| Total Carbohydrate | 47 | 50 |
| Total fat | 33 | 35 |
| | | |
| Fat proportions ... | | |
| Saturated fatty acids | 10 | 11 |
| Polyunsaturated fatty acids | 6 | 6.5 |
| Trans fatty acids | 2 | 2 |
| Monosaturated fatty acids | 12 | 13 |

*Alcohol should provide no more than 5% of energy in the diet.*

The Committee also suggested that the average intake of fibre, within a conventional food diet, should be 18g/day (individual range 12-24g/day) for adults.

## Energy

Energy is most often measured in calories, both for food and drink (calories consumed) and the energy used by the body to function (calories expended). *1 calorie is the amount of energy needed to increase the temperature of 1g of water by 1 degree centigrade.* Because the calorie is an extremely small unit, most people tend to use **kilocalorie** (1000 calories) when referring to measurements of the energy value of food.

The international equivalent of kilocalorie is the kilojoule, and you will find both values quoted on food labels. Kilocalories are sometimes called Calories, with a capital C, or abbreviated to kcal. See box above for conversion details.

The food we eat is made up of various chemical building blocks, each of which affects the body in different ways. These are carbohydrates, protein, fat, fibre, vitamins and minerals – all described below.

The calorific contents (per gram) of each of these elements is shown in the box, right.

| Calories per gram | |
|---|---|
| Protein | 4 |
| Carbohydrate | 4 |
| Fat | 9 |
| Alcohol | 7 |
| Vitamins, Minerals | 0 |
| Trace elements | 0 |
| Fibre | 0 |

## Protein

Protein is made up from 'building bricks' known as aminoacids. Altogether there are twenty-two, of which eight are essential. These are: Isoleucine, Leucine, Lysine, Methionine, Phenylalanine, Threonine, Tryptophan and Valine. If the diet does not contain enough of the 'essential' aminoacids, protein cannot be made in the body and its tissue eventually wastes away. Proteins provide the basic structural compounds of living cells. They are mostly found in the muscle tissue and the remainder in soft tissues such as liver, kidney and lung and also in teeth, blood and other fluids.

Protein is being continually made and destroyed. If the diet does not contain adequate protein, severe damage will occur to vital organs.

## Fat

Although the body contains a lot of fat (and in overweight people, too much), the amount of fat needed in the diet is very small, being just a few grams of essential fatty acids (EFA). The chief of these is linoleic acid. A deficiency of EFA is difficult to produce in man but in other animals a skin rash and anaemia is seen. EFA is important for the production of the prostaglandins, which are important substances in the body which regulate blood pressure, heart rate and the function of nerves.

## Carbohydrate

Besides fat, carbohydrate is the main source of energy in our diet. It is stored in the liver and muscles as glycogen for short-term energy requirements. Carbohydrates, or chemicals derived from them, are important constituents of cells, connective tissue and nerves, and in the liver they remove toxic products. When the carbohydrate in the diet is low (or absent), fat cannot be burned up completely and substances called 'ketones' are formed. These can be used by the brain instead of glucose. When ketones accumulate in the blood, 'ketosis' is said to develop. A mild 'ketosis' is not harmful and people may experience a feeling of 'euphoria' (or happiness). Since muscle protein can be broken down and converted into carbohydrates, a deficiency never occurs and there is no RDA. Carbohydrates also retain electrolytes in the body.

## Vitamins

Vitamins are a group of chemical compounds which are needed in only minute quantity and which are essential for the proper functioning of the body.

### Vitamin A

Also known as retinol – an essential component of the retina of the eye, and important in bone and skin growth. A deficiency causes 'night blindness'. High levels of vitamin A are toxic.

## Vitamin B1

Known also as thiamine, this is an essential part of an enzyme system necessary for the breakdown of carbohydrate. B1 deficiency causes a disease called 'beri-beri', which is characterized by weakness, numbness in the legs, and paralysis.

## Vitamin B2

Also known as riboflavin, this vitamin is also extremely important in key enzyme systems in the breakdown of carbohydrates and fat. A deficiency is characterized by cracks in the skin, and eye disease.

## Niacin or Nicotinamide)

An important component of several enzyme systems and necessary for the breakdown of fat and carbohydrate. A deficiency leads to the disease 'pellagra', characterized by weakness, fatigue, and ulceration of the mouth and tongue.

## Vitamin B6

Also known as pyridoxine, and needed in many enzyme systems, particularly those involved in the breakdown of protein. A deficiency leads to skin disease and anaemia.

## Pantothenic Acid

An essential part of an important enzyme system, this functions in the synthesis and breakdown of carbohydrates, proteins and fats. Experimental deficiency in man produces a wide variety of symptoms, particularly depression, fainting, rapid pulse and susceptibility to infection.

## Biotin

An important component of enzyme systems, involving the breakdown of fats and aminoacids. The deficiency is difficult to produce in man and animals. The chief abnormality is skin disease.

## Folic Acid

Involved in the formation of DNA and RNA, important constituents of all cells. A deficiency causes a special type of anaemia, in which the red cells are immature.

## Vitamin B12

Also called cyanocobalamin, this is essential for all cells, especially those of the gastrointestinal tract, bone marrow and nervous tissue. As with folic acid, a deficiency of B12 leads to anaemia caused by immaturity of the red cells. In addition, the function of the nervous system is affected.

## Vitamin C

Also known as ascorbic acid, this is needed for the normal function of cells. It is especially important in the adrenal gland, and the production and maintenance of collagen, a substance found in all fibrous tissue. It is abundant in the white cells of the blood, and thought to be important in the prevention of infection. A deficiency of Vitamin C leads to scurvy, which is characterized by skin haemorrhages, bleeding gums, and pains in the joints.

## Vitamin D

Another name for this is cholecaliferol. It is essential for the formation of bones and teeth and influences the absorption and use of calcium and phosphorus. A deficiency causes rickets in children, in which normal bone is not formed, and osteoporosis, a rarefaction of the bones in the elderly. Vitamin D can be made in the body by the action of sunlight on the skin. In large doses it is toxic.

## Vitamin E

Also called tocopherol, of which a number of forms exist (alphatocopherol is the most important). It is a strong antioxidant and prevents the oxidation of unsaturated fatty acids, especially essential fatty acids. In deficiency states, there is an increased tendency for the red cells to become unstable and break up. Nowadays, the vitamin is synthesized as alphatocopherol acetate.

In some varieties of the Cambridge Diet (for instance in the United Kingdom), extra vitamin E is added as an antioxidant, to prevent the small quantity of fat going rancid.

## Vitamin K

Also known as menadione, this is required for the normal production of an enzyme in the blood called prothrombin, essential for blood clotting. A deficiency leads to an increased tendency to bleed, and haemorrhage; this is very unlikely to happen because bacteria make the vitamin in the intestine. In large amounts it is toxic.

## Minerals

These are elements which are required by the body in relatively large amounts, and which are important in its structure and function.

## Calcium

The most abundant mineral in the body, since it is a major component, together with phosphorus, in the skeleton, It is also an important constituent of body fluids, especially the blood, where it is used in a large number of biochemical processes, such as blood clotting, nerve transmission, and regulation of the heart beat. A deficiency results in a tendency to develop rickets and osteomalacia. Together with vitamin D, it is all-important in preventing these.

## Phosphorus

Especially associated with calcium in the skeleton and in the body fluids. It is extremely important in many biochemical processes and is especially involved in the formation of DNA, RNA and phospholipids, which are key components of all cells. Like calcium, phosphorus is needed for the formation of healthy bones. An important point is that the ratio of calcium to phosphorus in the diet should be 1:1.

## Magnesium

An important constituent of bone, magnesium is a major constituent of fluid outside cells, and activates many enzymes. Magnesium deficiency can result in tetany (convulsions, cramps and muscle twitching), muscular weakness, and vertigo.

### Minerals

These are elements which are required by the body in relatively large amounts, and which are important in its structure and function:

- calcium
- phosphorous
- magnesium
- potassium
- sodium
- chloride
- sulphur

## Potassium

Most of the body's potassium is found inside the cells of the body, especially in muscle. It functions in regulating pH and the osmotic pressure of cells. It is necessary for the breakdown of carbohydrates and protein. A dietary deficiency can cause abnormal rhythm of the heart beats, and death from heart failure. Diuretics used for the treatment of high blood pressure often cause the elimination of potassium in the urine, and when potassium intake is low or restricted, the normal functioning of the heart may be adversely affected.

## Sodium

Surprisingly, about 30-45 per cent of the body's sodium is present in bone. It is a major component of the fluid surrounding cells and regulates pH, the osmotic pressure, and the amount of fluid in the body. It is difficult, if not impossible, to produce a dietary deficiency, since the body responds to lack by reducing its excretion. However, after a long period without sodium, a normal intake can lead to oedema – an accumulation of water in the joints. A high intake of sodium has been implicated in causing high blood pressure. There is no RDA of sodium but a moderately low intake is 1.5g, a low intake is less than 0.75g.

## Chloride

A component of the fluid surrounding cells, this activates enzymes, is involved in the maintenance of osmotic pressure, and is necessary for the breakdown of carbohydrates and protein, it is important in digestion, being part of the hydrochloric acid in the stomach. A deficiency can only occur when the body loses large amounts, as in vomiting, diarrhoea or sweating.

## Sulphur

The bulk of the sulphur in the body is in the sulphur-containing aminoacids. Although it is needed for metabolism, a deficiency of sulphur never occurs.

## Trace Elements

These are required by the body in very small amounts, and are important in its structure and function, particularly the latter.

### *Iron*

Most iron is found in the red cells as haemoglobin but it is important in the transfer of oxygen and in several enzyme systems. A deficiency leads to anaemia.

### *Zinc*

Present in most tissues, including muscle and bone, zinc is an important constituent of insulin and many enzymes, including those affecting immunity. A deficiency in man produces anaemia, poor growth, loss of hair, skin disease and a deficiency of male hormones.

### *Iodine*

> ## Trace Elements
>
> Only required in very small amounts. Important in its structure and (particularly) function:
>
> - iron
> - zinc
> - iodine
> - copper
> - manganese
> - flourine
> - selenium
> - molybdenum
> - cobalt
> - chromium

This element is a constituent of the thyroid hormone synthesized in the thyroid gland, which controls the release of total energy in the body. A deficiency of iodine leads to goitre in which the thyroid gland enlarges.

### *Copper*

Found in the body tissues including liver, brain, heart and kidney, copper is involved in several enzyme systems. There is no evidence that copper deficiency can occur in man.

### *Manganese*

This is found in bone and several of' the body tissues, and is important in enzyme systems, especially the liver. A deficiency has never been seen.

### *Fluorine*

Present in bone, fluorine reduces dental caries. Otherwise its nutritional importance is obscure. There is no RDA. Sufficient is now added to most drinking water or special toothpaste.

### *Selenium*

An important component of' an enzyme acting as an antioxidant. It functions in concert with vitamin E to protect the cells against hydrogen peroxide formation.

### *Molybdenum*

This element is important in at least two enzyme processes.

## Cobalt

The important constituent of vitamin B12. Enough cobalt is provided if there is sufficient B12 in the diet.

## Chromium

The function of this element is obscure but it appears to be involved in the breakdown of glucose. A deficiency produces diabetes.

## Fibre

This is material which is undigested by the body and which is for the most part excreted. Nutritionists now believe that it is much more important than hitherto recognized in the prevention of intestinal disease, and possibly in preventing many others.

## An Adequate and Balanced Diet

For many people, food is an important pleasure in life. It is also an important source of health and well-being. A single perfect food for ever would be boring and it is essential to eat a combination of a wide variety of different sorts of food: a balanced diet. A balanced diet contains the appropriate levels of protein, carbohydrate, fats, vitamins and minerals. Since most people do not accurately calculate what they eat, it is easier for consumers to have a guide to eating based on the recommended proportions of these types of food.

Some years ago, the Department of Health in the UK published 'The Balance of Good Health' to help people understand and enjoy healthy eating. It established Eight Guidelines for a Healthy Diet which are shown in the panel on the right. These principles are sound in other countries where specific foods may vary, but the food groups remain the same.

The 'The Balance of Good Health' also identified five food groups which are defined below and illustrated in the panel below, together with an indication of recommended relative proportion of each food group: about one-third from starchy foods found in bread and cereals, and another third from fruit and vegetables, for example. By choosing foods from each group in the right proportions, all the necessary nutrients to maintain health can be obtained. The five groups are described below, together with the recommended number of daily servings.

| Food Groups | | | |
|---|---|---|---|
| **Group** | **Description** | | **Proportion** |
| 1 | bread and cereals | pasta, rice, potatoes, noodles etc | 30% |
| 2 | fruit & vegetables | fresh, frozen and canned included | 30% |
| 3 | meat & fish | meat, poultry, fish, eggs, nuts etc | 15% |
| 4 | milk & dairy | milk, cheese, yoghurt etc | 15% |
| 5 | fat & sugar | margarine, butter, oils etc | 10% |

## Bread, other cereals and potatoes

Other cereals means things like breakfast cereals, pasta, rice, oats, noodles, maize, millet and cornmeal. Beans and pulses can be eaten as part of this group. These foods provide the 'bulk' of our diet and wholegrain varieties tend to contain the highest quantity of fibre, vitamins and minerals. The recommended daily intake of fibre is 18g for an adult.

**Provides** – Carbohydrate (starch); Fibre; Some calcium and iron; B vitamins

*Servings*

Between 5 and 11 servings a day: bread (1 slice), roll, breakfast cereal, potato (1 medium), rice, pasta or grains (50g). Choose wholegrain or high fibre options whenever you can

## Fruit and vegetables

Fresh, frozen and canned fruit and vegetables and dried fruit. A glass of fruit juice can also contribute. Beans and pulses can be eaten as part of this group.

Research continues to show that there are significant benefits from both the fibre and vitamin content of this group of foods – in particular the potential role of the anti-oxidant nutrients, vitamins A, C and E in protecting against cancer and heart disease. Intake of ACE vitamins can be ensured by having at least one green vegetable and one yellowy orange fruit or vegetable a day.

The UK's Department of Health have recently launched a '5-a-day' campaign to encourage people to eat at least 5 portions of a variety of fruit and vegetables each day, based on World Health organization recommendations.

**Provides** – Vitamin C; Carotenes; Folates; Fibre (NSP) and some carbohydrate

*Servings*

Eat at least five different servings of fruit and vegetables each day: fresh, frozen, canned, dried, and juices – see below for details of portion sizes. One portion of beans /pulses can also be counted in 5-a-Day

## Milk and dairy foods

Milk, cheese, yoghurt and fromage frais. This group does not include butter, eggs and cream. This group is essential for providing easily absorbed calcium, which is important for the strong development and maintenance of bones and teeth throughout life. It is especially important for young people and for breast-feeding mums.

**Provides** – Calcium, Zinc; Protein; Vitamin B12, B2; Vitamins A and D

*Servings:*

Between 2 and 4 servings a day: eg milk (200ml/7oz), cheese (small piece), yoghurt or fromage frais (small pot) and cottage cheese (100g/4oz). Choose low fat versions whenever you can.

## Meat, fish and alternatives

Meat, poultry, fish, eggs, nuts, beans and pulses as well as vegetarian alternatives such as quorn and soya protein.

These foods are the main source of protein in the diet – important for building and repairing body tissue. Meats are also the most easily available source of iron – essential for the formation of red blood cells. They also contain many of the B vitamins, zinc and magnesium. Beans (including baked beans) and lentils are a good source of fibre.

Oily fish are a good source of vitamin A and essential fatty acids, and at least one portion should be eaten per week. Preference should be given to oily fish (for example: salmon, herrings, mackerel, sardines), since it has been found in clinical trials that fish oil can reduce the incidence of coronary heart disease.

Although this group does include bacon, salami and meat products (such as sausages, beefburgers and paté), these are all relatively high fat choices, so should only be eaten occasionally and cooked without additional fat..

**Provides** – Iron; Protein; B Vitamins, especially B12; Zinc; Magnesium

*Servings:*

Between 1 and 3 servings a day of lean cut meat, poultry, fish or, if you are a vegetarian, peas, beans, lentils, nuts, or seeds. Quorn or tofu are a good vegetarian source of protein. Remove skin from poultry, trim fat off meat and cook with the minimum of additional fat.

## Foods containing fat and foods containing sugar

Foods containing fat: Margarine, butter, other spreading fats and low fat spreads, cooking oils, oil-based salad dressings, mayonnaise, cream, chocolate, crisps, biscuits, pastries, cake, puddings, ice-cream, rich sauces and gravies. Foods containing sugar: Soft drinks, sweets, jam and sugar as well as foods such as cake, puddings, biscuits, pastries and ice-cream.

Be aware of visible and hidden fats (see p7). As we saw above, average daily intake of fat should not exceed 33% of our total energy and saturated fatty acids should account for no more than 10%. Following this recommendation alone would not only help to reduce the incidence of heart disease but would help everyone maintain a healthy weight and reduce the increasing incidence of obesity.

Sugar is of little nutritional value and its use is discouraged: use fruit whenever possible.

**Provides** – Fat, including some essential fatty acids, but also limited amounts of Vitamin A and D. Most products also contain salt or sugar.

*Servings:*

Eat these foods sparingly: not very often and/or in small amounts.

## The Cambridge Diet Compared with Other Food

The food guide described above is the one most widely used by dietitians. There have, however, been many criticisms of it. When it was designed, the RDAs for certain nutrients such as phosphorus, iodine, vitamins B6, B12, E and K, folic acid, pantothenic acid, biotin and trace elements were not considered. Thus, while an individual can eat the correct number of servings, certain minerals may still be lacking, especially iron. It is a fallacy to suppose that by advising people to 'eat a wide variety of foods' all the requirements will be met, since no one can adequately define 'a wide variety of foods'. Some foods add many calories but no nutrients, others give large amounts of nutrients and few calories. Without a computer it is virtually impossible to choose a wide-ranging selection of food that does contain everything the body needs.

The great advantage of the Cambridge Diet is that it is a nutritionally dense and balanced food. In a small number of calories, every nutrient is included in just the right amounts. This is particularly reassuring to someone who is busy, and does not have the time to work out the nutrient content of a diet from food tables.

# Calorie Controlled Recipes 16

The recipes in this chapter were designed to complement the Cambridge programmes, from 1000 kcal upwards. Each recipe includes an indication of the 'fat gram' content. This is shown in square brackets – eg [5g]. Remember that 1g of fat equals 9kcal, compared to only 4kcal per gram for protein and carbohydrate. Therefore, we recommend that those on the 1000 kcal programme do not exceed 35 fat grams a day in your choices – keep to 50 fat grams on the 1200 kcal programme.

> ### In these recipes
>
> 1 large slice wholemeal bread is about 40g (1½oz)
> 1 small wholemeal roll is 50g (2oz)
> tsp = standard measure teaspoon = 5ml
> tbsp = standard measure tablespoon = 15ml
> (**V**) = suitable for vegetarians

## Breakfasts

### 50 kcal [0g]
Large wedge of melon *(V)*
l00g (4oz) stewed apple sweetened with artificial sweetener and topped with 2 tbsp natural yoghurt.
1 small banana – 75g (3oz) peeled weight
125g pot diet yoghurt.
2 canned pineapple rings in natural juice, topped with 2 tbsp low fat natural yoghurt.
1 orange, 1 apple, 1 pear, 2 satsumas, 1 peach, 1 nectarine, ½ fresh mango or 75g (3oz) grapes

### 150 kcal
1 medium banana – 125g (4½oz) peeled weight – sliced and topped with 125g pot diet yoghurt [1g].
½ grapefruit and 1 orange – segmented – and topped with 100g (4oz) very low fat fromage frais and 2 tsp honey [0g].
2 Weetabix, milk from allowance and 1 tbsp raisins [0g -2g with semi-skimmed milk].

25g (1oz) muesli, milk from allowance topped with 1 sliced nectarine or peach 2g – 4g when using semi-skimmed milk]

50ml (½ pint) unsweetened orange juice; 1 large slice wholemeal toast with 1 tsp low fat spread and 1 tsp pure fruit spread [5g].

1 (size 3) boiled egg with 1 Ryvita and 1tsp low fat spread [7g].

## 250 kcal

½ grapefruit and 1 orange segmented and topped with 150g pot natural low fat yogurt; 1 large slice wholemeal toast with 1 tsp low fat spread and 1 tsp pure fruit spread [6g].

1 Weetabix with milk from allowance, topped with 3 tsp very low fat fromage frais; 1 large slice wholemeal toast with 1 tsp low fat spread and 1 tsp pure fruit spread [5g – 7g with semi-skimmed milk].

2 large slices wholemeal toast with 2 tsp low fat spread and 1 small banana 75g (3oz) peeled weight [10g].

1 (size 3) boiled egg and 2 large slices wholemeal toast cut into fingers with 1 tsp low fat spread [8g].

1 wholemeal roll with 1 tsp low fat spread and 2 tsp marmalade; 1 satsuma; 125g pot diet yogurt [6g].

## 300 kcal

½ grapefruit; 2 (size 3) eggs scrambled with a little milk from allowance and cooked with ½ tsp margarine to grease the pan, served on 1½ large slices wholemeal toast [10g] (V)

25g (1oz) Bran Flakes with milk from allowance; 2 large slices wholemeal toast with 2 tsp low fat spread topped with 2 sliced tomatoes, grilled [10g – 12g with semi-skimmed milk] (V)

2 large slices wholemeal bread spread with 1 tsp margarine, filled with 50g (2oz) half fat edam, cooked in a sandwich toaster or grilled [16g] (V)

1 grilled low fat sausage, 1 (size 3) poached egg and 2 grilled tomatoes with 1 large slice wholemeal bread and 1 tsp low fat spread [15g].

2 grilled rashers lean back bacon, trimmed of fat, with 1 (size 3) poached egg and 1 slice wholemeal bread and 1 tsp low fat spread [17g].

Porridge made with 25g (1oz) oats, 200m1 (7f1oz) milk from allowance and 3 tsp sugar; 1½ large slices wholemeal toast with 1½ tsp low fat spread and 1½ tsp pure fruit spread [7g – 10g with semi-skimmed milk] (V)

## Starters

## 50 kcal

Large wedge of melon [0g] (V)

300ml (10 floz) consommé [0g]

1 serving 50 kcal soup – check your local supermarket for availability [0g] (V)

Tomato and onion salad – slice 2 tomatoes and top with 1 tbsp mild chopped onion and freshly ground black pepper, garnish with 1 tbsp chopped parsley and 4 black olives, serve with oil free French dressing [3g] (V)

225g (8oz) fresh asparagus, steamed and served with 1 tsp low fat spread [6g](V)

100g (4oz) button mushrooms cooked in enough tomato juice to cover, seasoned with 1 tbsp tomato purée, chopped fresh herbs and a pinch paprika [1g] (V)

## 60 to 75 kcal

Slice the top from 1 small tomato, scoop out the seeds and discard. Fill with 25g (1oz) cottage cheese with sweetcorn and peppers mixed with a few shelled prawns. Garnish with a couple of prawns [1g].

Serve ½ grapefruit and 1 orange, filleted and garnished with a mint leaf [0g] *(V)*

Arrange a bed of sliced iceberg lettuce on a plate. Top with grated carrot. Arrange on top 2 sliced tomatoes, a little chopped onion, a little chopped green or red pepper and 1 tablespoon sweetcorn kernels. Pour over a little oil free vinaigrette dressing [1g] *(V)*

Place half a hard boiled egg on a bed of water cress with 50g (2oz) sliced mushrooms, and top with 2 teaspoons low calorie mayonnaise mixed with fresh chopped mixed herbs [5g] *(V)*

## 150 kcal

75g (3oz) rollmop herring served with lettuce, cucumber and 1 tomato [9g].

225g (8oz) corn on the cob served with 1tsp low fat spread [7g] *(V)*

Arrange a bed of shredded lettuce in a glass sundae dish or on a small plate, top with 50g (2oz) peeled prawns and 2 tbsp low calorie tomato or seafood dressing, serve with a 25g (1oz) slice wholemeal bread and a scraping of low fat spread [4g].

Arrange a bed of shredded lettuce on a small plate and top with 1 sliced tomato, some chopped onion, 50g (2oz) cooked French beans, 50g (2oz) tuna canned in brine, drained and flaked, a (size 5) sliced hard boiled egg, 2 anchovy fillets and 2 black olives, served with oil free French dressing [8g].

## Lunches

## 300 kcal

50g (2oz) hunk wholemeal French bread cut open, filled with 50g (2oz) curd cheese, sliced tomato, watercress sprigs and some sliced cucumber; 1 orange [8g] *(V)*

2 large slices wholemeal bread spread with 2 tsp low fat spread, 2 tsp pure fruit spread and filled with a sliced banana, 125g (4½oz) peeled weight [10g]*(V)*

1 can calorie-reduced soup (up to 70 kcal), with 1 wholemeal roll, 2 tsp low fat spread; 1 apple [10g] *(V)*

1 large slice wholemeal bread with 1 tsp low fat spread, topped with shredded lettuce, 1 tbsp low calorie salad cream, 75g (3oz) sliced lean ham, some sliced cucumber, tomato and spring onion; 5 stewed prunes [9g].

1 small Scotch egg, weighing 100g (4oz), with a salad of lettuce, radish, celery, tomato, cucumber, watercress, chicory and spring onions; ½ a fresh mango [18g].

1 granary roll cut open, spread with 1 tsp low fat spread and filled with 40g (1½ oz) sliced low fat Cheddar and some sliced cucumber; 1 satsuma [11g] *(V)*

## 350 kcal

2 large slices wholemeal bread with 2 tsp low fat spread filled with 1 sliced hard boiled egg and 2 tsp low calorie mayonnaise; 1 pear [17g] *(V)*

2 large slices wholemeal toast topped with 150g (5oz) sugar free baked beans and 25g (1oz) grated low fat Cheddar [6g].

100g (4oz) pot cottage cheese and chives, with 1 large grated carrot, 1 sliced tomato, 1 celery stalk, and 1 wholemeal mini pitta bread; 75g (3oz) grapes [5g] *(V)*

2 large slices wholemeal toast topped with 50g (2oz) grated low fat Cheddar, a little chopped onion and a sliced tomato, grilled until the cheese has melted, serve with 1 tsp tomato and chilli relish; 125g pot diet yogurt [10g] *(V)*

Spread 2 slices of wholemeal bread from a small sliced loaf with 2 teaspoons low fat spread. Sandwich with 30g (1.25oz) grated half fat Cheddar, 25g (1oz) lean ham and 1 ring pineapple (tinned in natural juice and drained on absorbent kitchen paper). Cook under the grill or in a toasted sandwich maker, serve with 1 grilled tomato and a large green salad with oil free vinaigrette dressing [16g].

1 low fat burger, grilled and served in 1 burger bun with 1 tomato sliced, and sliced gherkin; 1 peach and 150g pot low fat raspberry yogurt [10g].

### 450 kcal

75g (3oz) hunk wholemeal French bread with 2 tsp low fat spread, 40g (1½oz) hunk low fat Cheddar, 1 tbsp piccalilli, 2 pickled onions, sliced tomato, lettuce and cucumber; 1 apple [17g] *(V)*

2 large slices wholemeal bread with 2 tsp low fat spread, filled with shredded lettuce, 105g can pink salmon, skin and bones removed and flaked, and 1 tsp low calorie mayonnaise; 1 pear and 125g diet yogurt [17g].

215g can ravioli in tomato sauce served on 2 large slices wholemeal toast and topped with 25g (1oz) grated low fat Cheddar with 1 grilled tomato; 1 apple [10g].

Grill two large low fat sausages and serve with ½ a 450g tin of reduced-calorie baked beans and 2 grilled tomatoes [8g].

225g (8oz) baked potato split and filled with 50g (2oz) brie cheese, and served with sliced iceberg lettuce, cress and 125g pot calorie reduced coleslaw; 2 canned apricot halves in natural juice with 2 tbsp natural low fat yogurt [19g] *(V)*

3 large slices wholemeal bread with 3 tsp low fat spread filled with 75g (3oz) roast chicken, lettuce and cucumber; 2 satsumas [17g].

2 rollmop herrings with a wedge of lemon, served with 1 slice of pumpernickel bread spread with 1 tsp low fat spread, sliced tomato, cucumber, shredded lettuce, 1 grated carrot, a little chopped pepper and 1 spring onion; 1 peach [24g].

## Main Courses

### 300 kcal per serving

#### Tandoori Fish Bake

Mix 1 tablespoon tandoori paste with 1 tablespoon natural yoghurt. Pour over 225g (8oz) haddock or whiting fillet in a dish, cover and refrigerate for 4 hours or overnight. Bake at 180degC (350F, Gas Mark 4) for 20 to 30 minutes. Serve with 2 tablespoons cooked rice and 50g (2oz) poached mushrooms [3g].

#### Stuffed Mushrooms

Remove stalks from 2 large field mushrooms and cook them under a slow grill. Fill them with Mushroom Savoury Rice (proprietary brand), cook according to instructions. Top with 50g (2oz) grated half fat Edam, and return to the grill to allow the cheese to melt. Serve with a large green salad with oil free vinaigrette dressing. [11g] *(V)*

*Easy Chicken Casserole (Serves 2, 6g fat per serving)*

Remove the skin from 4 chicken thighs and place them in a casserole dish. Pour over 4 tablespoons red wine and 390g tin of tomatoes, and add 100g (4oz) each of chopped courgette, aubergine and onion. Cover and bake at 180degC (350F, Gas Mark 4) for 35 to 40 minutes. Serve with 200g (7oz) cooked French beans and 200g (7oz) cauliflower [6g].

## 300 – 350 kcal per serving

*Broccoli in Cheese and Mushroom Sauce*

Make a cheese and mushroom sauce by placing 15g (½oz) low fat spread, 15g (½oz) plain flour, 150 ml (qtr pint) skimmed milk and 50g (2oz) chopped mushrooms in a saucepan and whisking together over a medium heat until the sauce has thickened. Stir in 25g (1oz) grated Parmesan cheese. Pour over 100g (4oz) cooked broccoli florets and serve with a grilled beef tomato [16g](V)

*Cheese Omelette*

Beat 2 size 3 eggs with 1 tablespoon skimmed milk and a pinch of mixed herbs. Cook in an omelette pan with 1 teaspoon oil. Add 25g (1oz) sliced half fat Edam to the omelette. Fold over when it has set and serve with a salad of lettuce, shredded red cabbage, 2 tomatoes, carrot, cucumber, radish, watercress and onion tossed with oil free vinaigrette dressing [20g] (V)

*Baked Potato and Tzatziki or Cottage Cheese*

Fill a 225g (8oz) baked potato with 150g (5oz) tzatziki (or 113 g pot half fat cottage cheese), and serve with a salad of grated carrot, tomato, cucumber, lettuce and watercress with oil free vinaigrette dressing [8g] (V)

*Pork Escalope with Chips*

Grill 100g (4oz) lean pork escalope and serve with 75g (3oz) oven chips and 2 grilled tomatoes [8g].

*Egg and Cheese Salad*

Serve 1 hard boiled egg with 50g (2oz) grated half fat Edam, a large salad of lettuce, watercress, 2 tomatoes, cucumber, shredded red cabbage, chopped onion and chopped green pepper tossed in oil free vinaigrette dressing, 50g (2oz) calorie reduced coleslaw and 1 small slice wholemeal bread – 25g (1oz) – with 1 teaspoon low fat spread [20g] (V)

*Omelette*

1 omelette made with 2 (size 3) eggs using ½ tsp margarine to grease the pan, filled with 25g (1oz) grated low fat Cheddar and 1 sliced button mushroom, served with 40g (1½oz) dry weight cooked wholewheat pasta shapes and 100g (4oz) broccoli [21g] (V)

*Smoked Mackerel Salad*

Serve 100g (4oz) smoked mackerel fillet with 1 grated carrot, 1 tomato, sliced cucumber, watercress and 50g (2oz) calorie-reduced potato salad [22g].

## 400 kcal

### Spicy Turkey

150g (5oz) turkey breast fillet, brushed with chilli and garlic sauce and grilled, served with 200g (7oz) canned ratatouille and 40g (1½oz) dry weight cooked brown rice [6g].

### Savoury Chicken

2 chicken thighs, skinned, brushed with soy sauce and grilled, served with 100g (4oz) cooked spinach, 40g (1½oz) dry weight cooked brown rice, 50g (2oz) poached mushrooms and 2tbsp tomato and chilli relish [7g].

### Grilled Steak

100g (4oz) lean steak, grilled, 100g (4oz) oven chips, 50g (2oz) peas, 2 grilled tomatoes, 50g (2oz) poached mushrooms lightly cooked in stock [10g].

### Bacon Steaks

100g (4oz) grilled bacon steak, served with 100g (4oz) peas, 100g (4oz) oven chips and 150g (5oz) sugar free baked beans [10g].

### Poached Haddock

225g (8oz) poached haddock, served with 225g (8oz) boiled potatoes, 175g (6oz) canned tomatoes and 50g (2oz) poached mushrooms [2g].

### Grilled Trout

175g (6oz) trout grilled, with 1 tbsp tartare sauce, 175g (6oz) baked potato, topped with 1 tsp low fat spread and a little fresh chopped parsley, served with 100g (4oz) broccoli and 100g (4oz) carrots [14g].

### Savoury Jacket Potato with Tuna

225 (8oz) baked potato, split and filled with 40g (1½oz) grated low fat Cheddar cheese and 100g (4oz) tuna canned in brine, drained and flaked [7g].

### Stir Fry Pork with Peppers

Heat 1 tablespoon oil in a wok or large frying pan and cook 1 sliced spring onion, one inch piece grated root ginger and 2 crushed garlic cloves for 30 to 45 seconds. Add 100g (4oz) finely sliced pork escalope or other cut of lean pork and cook for 2 minutes. Add 2 sliced celery stalks, a sliced green pepper, 50g (2oz) mushrooms, a pinch of Chinese 'five-spice' powder, 1 tablespoon soy sauce and 1 tablespoon dry sherry and cook for a further 1½ to 2 minutes. Serve with 50g (2oz) dry weight egg thread noodles, cooked in boiling water [20g].

# Desserts

## *50 kcal [all 0g]*

100g (4oz) stewed apple sweetened with artificial sweetener and topped with 2 tbsp natural yoghurt.

1 small banana, 75g (3oz) peeled weight 125g pot diet yoghurt.

2 canned pineapple rings in natural juice topped with 2 tbsp low fat natural yoghurt.

1 orange, 1 apple, 1 pear, 2 satsumas, 1 peach, 1 nectarine, 75g (3oz) grapes or ½ fresh mango

## *70 kcal*

Drain and sieve 300g (10oz) tin blackcurrants in natural juice. Mix into ½of a 425g tin low fat custard and stir in 100g (4oz) thick Greek yoghurt. (Serves 6 – 1g fat per serving) [1g].

Fruit salad made with 1 sliced apple, 1 segmented orange, 1 sliced kiwi fruit, 100g (4oz) strawberries, 100g (4oz) seedless grapes, ½ melon – cubed, 1 sliced pear, 225g tin pineapple cubes in natural juice and 150ml unsweetened orange juice. (Serves 6) [0g]

Press 100g (4oz) tinned raspberries in natural juice through a sieve and discard the seeds. Mix the fruit purée with 1 tablespoon natural yoghurt and serve over 100g (4oz) fresh strawberries or 1 sliced kiwi fruit [1g].

Peel and slice 1 pear, and poach in 150m1 (qtr pint) water with 100ml (3½floz) sweet cider with thin strips of orange rind. (Serves 2) [0g]

## *150 kcal*

150g pot low fat yogurt [1g]

100g (4oz) raspberries canned in natural juice topped with 100g (4oz) very low-fat fromage frais and 1 tbsp toasted almonds [7g].

1 meringue nest filled with ½ can fruit cocktail in fruit juice from 250g can, drained, topped with 2 tbsp very low fat fromage frais and 1 tbsp flaked almonds [7g].

225g (8oz) cooking apple cored, filled with 2 tsp raisins and 2 tsp demerara sugar and 1 tsp low fat spread and baked in a medium oven for 30 minutes [4g].

1 serving poached pear (see above), with 100g (4oz) very low fat fromage frais [0g]

50g (2oz) curd cheese mixed with 2 tsp pure fruit spread, served on ½ fresh pear [6g].

## Treats And Snacks

### Free Foods

cucumber, celery, lettuce, watercress, green pepper with oil free French dressing.

### 25 kcal

| | | |
|---|---|---|
| 1 large raw carrot [0g] | 1 small kiwi fruit [0g] | 1 satsuma [0g] |
| l brazil nut [2g] | 5 peanuts [2g] | 3 dried apricots [0g] |
| 2 glasses of low calorie squash [0g] | | 150m1 (qtr pint) tomato juice |
| [0g] | | |

### 50 kcal

| | | |
|---|---|---|
| 1 finger of Kit-Kat [2g] | 1 Jaffa cake [1g] | 1 ginger nut biscuit [2g] |
| 1 rich tea biscuit [1g] | 3 wine gums [0g] | 2 small toffees [2g] |

150m1 (qtr pint) unsweetened orange juice [0g]
150m1 (qtr pint) alcohol-free wine [0g]
275ml can/bottle alcohol-free lager [0g]

### 100 kcal

15g (½oz) sunflower seeds  [7g]
3 dried figs [1g]
40g (1½oz) raisins [0g]
40g (1½oz) hunk half fat edam with 1 tomato [5g]
1 mini wholemeal pitta bread [1g]
150m1 (qtr  pint) grape juice [0g]
1 large slice wholemeal bread with 1 tsp low fat spread [5g]
330ml can/bottle alcohol free lager 0g]

### 150 kcal

28g packet crisps [6g]
l jam tart [5g]
1 wholemeal roll with 1 tsp low fat spread [5g]
30g packet mixed nuts and raisins [12g]
225g (8oz) corn on the cob [3g]
150g (5oz) baked potato [0g]

### 200 kcal

1 currant bun with 2 tsp low fat spread [11g]
2 toasted crumpets with 2 tsp low fat spread [9g]
1 wholemeal roll with 1½ tsp low fat spread and 2 tsp honey [7g]
125g (4½oz) oven chips [5g]
1 wholemeal scone with 1 tsp low fat spread [3g]
50g (2oz) carrot cake [10g]

# Questions and Answers

# 17

At Cambridge we are often asked about our products and programmes as well as more general queries on nutrition, obesity etc. We have included the most frequent of these questions in a number of categories:

☐ Using the Cambridge Diet
☐ Using the Diet with Disorders
☐ Effects of the Diet
☐ Medical Queries
☐ Product information
☐ Weight Loss with the Diet
☐ General Nutrition

## Using the Cambridge Diet

### *How much water should I drink when on the Cambridge Diet?*

It is very important to consume at least eight glasses of water or other liquid per day. Since our bodies consist of over 60 per cent water, it is very important that we constantly replace our body fluids. Sufficient liquid intake is also necessary to maintain proper kidney function.

### *Why must I drink so much?*

There are several reasons. A good rule of thumb for good health is to drink 4pt (2.25 ltr) of fluid a day whether trying to lose weight or not. If the Cambridge Diet is used as the 'Sole Source' of nutrition, this is the minimum for good health – 6-8pt (3 to 4ltr) would be even better. The reasons for this include:

- A very low calorie diet (VLCD) like Cambridge produces a natural water loss and this must be replaced.
- Food is largely composed of water, just like our bodies. On the "Sole Source" programme it is necessary to compensate for the fluid that would otherwise have been taken in through food. It is important to keep the body's fluid levels topped up to prevent the unpleasant symptoms of dehydration – headache, dizziness, fatigue, irritability and constipation.
- The Cambridge Diet offers complete nutrition but in a very concentrated form. It is therefore ideal to have 250ml (½ pint) of water before each diet to dilute the concentration of minerals and to help prevent any possible feeling of nausea.
- Extra fluid enables the body to get rid of the waste products associated with the breakdown of fats resulting from weight loss.

## I don't like black tea and coffee – can I have low-calorie squashes?

Not on the "Sole Source" programme. Research has shown that citric acid can prevent the body utilising its carbohydrate stores and cause fluid retention. As citric acid is present in 'one calorie' diet drinks, low-calorie fruit squashes, slices of lemon and lemon tea, any of these may for some people negate the effectiveness of the Diet. It is possible to whiten tea and coffee using small amounts of vanilla flavoured Diet from the daily quota. Leaf herb teas (mint, nettle, etc) can add variety, but avoid fruit and flower teas as they contain small amounts of carbohydrate which can cause fluid retention and induce a plateau in some dieters. Those who cannot live without the daily enjoyment of tea and coffee with milk can still lose weight with Cambridge by following one of the "with food" programmes (see Chapter 2) for which there is a daily milk allowance.

## Is alcohol allowed while taking the Cambridge Diet as the sole source of nutrition?

No. Alcohol contains seven calories per gram and is of no other significant nutritional value.

## Is it all right to drink coffee while taking the Cambridge Diet as the sole source of nutrition?

Consumption of large quantities of coffee or Colas is not recommended. If you feel you must drink them, the decaffeinated forms are preferred. Caffeine acts as a stimulant to the body systems and sometimes provides an irritant effect. Herbal teas offer a pleasant alternative.

## Will I feel hungry when on 'Sole Source'?

Some hunger is experienced during the first one or two days but on the third day it usually disappears completely. This is because your body has adjusted to its new balance of just over 400 kcal per day. If you cheat, you will become very hungry indeed, because eating food only stimulates your hunger more, so it is best to stick to the Diet and do not supplement it, at least for four weeks when you can have a break.

## Can I chew calorie-free gum on the 'Sole Source' programme?

It is best not to because chewing gum stimulates the release of gastric juices which in turn will make you feel hungry. Only chew for 2 or 3 minutes if you feel you have to.

## Will I need vitamin supplements while using the Cambridge Diet?

The big plus about Cambridge is that, unlike other diets, you do not need to take extra supplements. Each item offers a third of the recommended daily allowance of all vitamins, minerals and trace elements, so three a day give complete nutrition. The main worry when people go on food-based slimming diets, is that reduction in food means reduced nutrient intake which in turn puts health at risk. It is impossible to achieve complete nutrition from conventional food on less than 1500 Kcal a day. Even then, extensive nutritional knowledge and a wide variety of foods need to be consumed to ensure adequate intake of all those vitamins and minerals. Cambridge has cracked that problem by formulating a diet that gives 100% nutrition and has programmes (up to 1500 kcal per day) using the Diet as a nutritional foundation with conventional food. Cambridge customers have confidence that they can lose weight safely and not put health at risk.

*Some days I feel completely satisfied with only two Cambridge Diet meals. Do I need to take the third meal?*

Yes. Three Cambridge meals provide all the necessary nutrients for one day to keep your body in a good nutritional state.

*If I am really hungry, can I take a fourth Cambridge Diet meal without spoiling my diet?*

Some people may require additional energy for their activities, such as those involved in heavy physical work and strenuous athletics. An extra Cambridge Diet meal may be necessary to provide extra energy in balanced form.

*At what age should a person refrain from taking the Cambridge Diet?*

A person who has medical problems should not be on any type of diet without a doctor's supervision. However, the Cambridge Diet Plan has helped extremely elderly people who have a problem with eating sufficient food to provide proper nutrition.

*Can a sixteen year old use any of the Cambridge Diet weight loss programmes?*

Yes, but not the "Sole Source" or 790 kcal programmes without their doctor's involvement. Children between the ages of 14 and 18 should be encouraged to follow healthy eating advice given in 'Balance of Good Health' (Health Education Authority) and to increase levels of activity. If this is unsuccessful, then a Cambridge programme with food (1000 to 1500 kcal) can be followed. The recommendations for this programme are very specific, carefully structured and easy to follow. The involvement of the child's parent or guardian should be encouraged wherever possible. If a lower calorie ("Sole Source" or 790 kcal) programme is specifically requested, then parental involvement is necessary, and the doctor should be consulted and kept informed of progress.

Young people require lots of support to keep them motivated, to ensure they follow the programme correctly and to achieve a realistic stable weight long term.

## *Do I need to prepare for the 'Sole Source' programme?*

Yes. Problems arising at the start of the 'Sole Source' programme can be prevented by preparing in the week prior to the agreed start date by:

* gradually reducing food intake, particularly carbohydrate. This will prevent carbohydrate withdrawal headaches and hasten the onset of ketosis with all its benefits – particularly reduced hunger.
* introducing a Cambridge Diet once or twice a day to help to reduce energy intake. This will result in reduced glycogen stores, ensuring the benefits of ketosis are enjoyed sooner rather than later.
* using a natural bulking agent (eg Fibre 89) at a level appropriate to your needs will prevent a problem later (for those who have a history of constipation).
* increasing water intake to 1.7 ltrs (3 pts) per day.
* checking with your doctor.

Preparation will prevent "The Last Supper Syndrome", ie a binge the day before 'Sole Source' which increases glycogen stores, delaying the onset of ketosis and increasing feelings of tiredness and hunger.

We recommend that you prepare for a week on the next step up from that selected for weight loss. For example, if it was agreed to follow the 790 kcal programme for weight loss, prepare at the 1000 kcal level, then drop down for the weight loss phase.

## When do I need to think about maintenance?

At the beginning. The importance of maintenance needs to be made clear to anyone embarking on a Cambridge weight loss programme at whatever calorific level. Weight maintenance does not start when target weight is achieved but should be a significant component of the initial consideration when the obese person first seeks help. Successful long term weight management is only achieved by making long-term permanent changes to diet and lifestyle. The seeds for these long term changes need to be sown early. Cambridge is not a "quick fix". The role of the Diet and the Cambridge Counsellor is ongoing.

## Once I reach target weight, how do I maintain it?

If a person achieves a desired weight and then goes back to the bad food habits of a lifetime that put the weight on in the first place, it is inevitable that the weight lost will be regained. The Cambridge Diet gives rapid weight-loss, but it also provides a sound nutritional base for those who are at their desired weight and who want to keep it. The method I recommend is that you will take your Cambridge Diet three times per day even when your desired weight is achieved. Along with this nutritional base you should then add one or two meals totalling 400 to 800 kcal until the scales show how many calories you can absorb and still maintain your desired weight.

## Do you recommend exercise with the Cambridge Diet?

Do not start a strenuous exercise programme at the same time as you start the Cambridge Diet. (IF you are already taking exercise then you may continue it.) Moderate exercise is useful once you start to lose weight, providing that it is approached with caution and not done with excess. Walking or cycling is excellent exercise, but start slowly, and do not overdo it at the beginning.

## I am a Muslim; how can I continue with the 'Sole Source' programme during Ramadan?

Ramadan occurs in the ninth month of the Muslim year. During daylight hours, rigid fasting is observed which means that Cambridge Diet and water will need to be consumed before sunrise and after sun-down. During the time available, intake should be spread out as evenly as possible and might necessitate rising a bit earlier. It is not advisable to take more than one diet at a time as the increased carbohydrate intake may take the customer out of ketosis, making it even more difficult for them to stay motivated and stick with the programme.

## Why is it recommended that people take 'Sole Source' for no more than four consecutive weeks?

This advice complies with the recommendations in the 1987 DHSS report by the Committee on the Medical Aspects of Food Policy (COMA) entitled 'The Use of Very Low Calorie Diets in Obesity': "As the Sole Source of nourishment, the use of VLCD should not exceed the period recommended by the manufacturers (up to 3 to 4 weeks at a time) without reverting to a normal mixture of foods". The above recommendation from COMA was not based on any research, but when the doctors who participated in Cambridge's clinical trials were asked what was the maximum time they would recommend the diet be used sole source, without medical supervision, the consensus of opinion was four weeks.

If you want to forego the 'Add-a-meal' week, you can only do so with your doctor's written consent.

I have been taking the Cambridge Diet as my sole source of nutrition for four weeks. What should I eat in the fifth "Add-a-meal" week?

Continue to have three Cambridge Diet meals a day and add a daily "green and white" meal (just under 400kcal). "Green" means a portion of leafy greens and vegetables. "White" could be portion of skinless lean chicken breast, grilled fish or cottage cheese. See Chapter 2 for a list of acceptable foods

## Using the Diet with Disorders

### I am under treatment for depression. Is it safe for me to take the Cambridge diet?

There is nothing in the Cambridge Diet plan that would interfere with depression therapy. It is important, however, that any diet you undergo be supervised very carefully by your doctor or psychiatrist.

I seem to have a recurring problem with heartburn and have an ulcer. Will the Cambridge Diet aggravate this condition?

On the contrary, the Cambridge Diet is easily digested, and reports indicate that it has a very soothing effect on the stomach. Some people swear that the Cambridge Diet drinks have reduced their symptoms drastically. It may be necessary to take six mini meals per day instead of the three regular Cambridge Diet meals, but the ingredients in the Cambridge Diet will not interfere with ulcers or ulcer medication. If you are on medication for ulcers, be sure to contact your doctor before going on any diet.

### I am on a low sodium diet. How much salt is there in Cambridge?

The Cambridge Diet contains approximately 500 mg of sodium per serving, or approximately 1,500 mg salt per day. A doctor should be consulted if the dieter has been placed on a low sodium diet, to make sure that the sodium intake is not in excess of the doctor's recommendation.

### I have a thyroid condition and am on medication. Can I safely take the Cambridge Diet?

The Cambridge Diet is compatible with all standard thyroid procedures, but I would recommend consulting your doctor before starting any diet.

### Can a person with diabetes be on the Cambridge Diet?

Many of my colleagues have found that by changing from three Cambridge Diet meals per day, to six mini meals the dieter's caloric intake is controlled. We have seen great success with diabetic patients using the Cambridge Diet. Diabetics are cautioned, however, not to embark on any diet programme without first consulting their physician. Those who have Diabetes Type 1 and are taking insulin are contraindicated (see Chapter 4)

### How does the Cambridge Diet affect those with hypoglycemia?

Hypoglycemia is the opposite of diabetes. Low blood sugar often results from poor nutrition. The Cambridge Diet made into six mini meals per day does an excellent job of keeping the blood sugar level in hypoglycemic people.

### I have raised cholesterol levels. Can I use the Cambridge Diet?

No problem. Studies have shown that using the Cambridge Diet as the sole source of nutrition cuts levels of blood cholesterol by an average of 25% and blood fats by an average of 40% – the reduction seems to be greatest in those with initial high levels. When patients returned to a normal diet levels rose again, but not as high as before. There is also some evidence that, following weight loss, ongoing use of the Diet as part of a healthy diet, ie with lots of fresh fruit and vegetables, cereals, lean meat, oily fish (eg salmon, herring, mackerel, etc), and unsaturated fats, could also help control cholesterol levels.

### Is a lactose intolerant three-year-old too young to enjoy a drink of lactose-free Cambridge Diet?

Over the years many a Counsellor's child or grandchild has enjoyed Cambridge Diet as a delicious milkshake drink. There is nothing in it that will cause harm and it is certainly more nutritious than many children's drinks. A half a portion at a time is enough for a small child, with a total of one whole Diet per day. This will probably be as much as she can drink and it would be a shame to waste it; and the level of nutrients will not be so concentrated. The same goes for lactose-free Cambridge Diet which is available in selected flavours.

### Does the Cambridge Diet help with the bowel disease Diverticulitis?

Diverticulosis is the development of diverticula (small sacs) in the bowel. Diverticulitis is a complication produced by inflammation of the diverticula. Symptoms can include bloating, pain in the lower abdomen, and changes in bowel habits. Lack of fibre may play a part in the development of this condition and a high fibre diet might reduce the incidence of complications. So how does dieting affect the condition? With any change in eating habits a change in bowel habits can follow. No two people are the same and there is no telling whether Cambridge will help or not. Initially, try six half portions. Or, try the higher-fibre 790 kcal programme.

### What is the advice for someone with a history of constipation?

Natural bulking agents should be used in the preparation week to ensure there are no existing problems at the start of the weight loss process. A change of eating habits will almost inevitably cause a change in bowel habits for everyone. 'Fibre 89' is a very effective natural bulking agent available only from Cambridge Health Plan. There are other over-the-counter remedies but it is becoming more difficult to obtain products that do not have added carbohydrate – which would undermine the 'Sole Source' programme. 'Fibre 89' is very economic – a 125g tub provides 40 servings. It is also very versatile as it can be mixed in any drink, hot or cold, and its presence remains undetected.

### Can people with high blood pressure take the Cambridge Diet for weight-loss and is it permissible to take diuretics?

Many people with high blood pressure have experienced extremely positive results taking the Cambridge Diet for weight-loss. Not only has there been a significant drop in blood pressure, but also a normalization which allowed a decrease in medication previously required. It is very important that these people consult their doctors, especially if they are taking medication. The Cambridge Diet, taken as a sole source of nutrition, will itself cause water loss. Any artificial diuretics added to the diet could seriously deplete your potassium balance and cause dizziness, weakness and fatigue. For this reason, medication having a diuretic effect should not be taken concurrently with the Cambridge Diet except with the approval of a doctor.

### I have high blood pressure. Can I use the Diet?

Yes. You can take the Cambridge Diet as a Sole Source of nutrition providing that your doctor agrees and signs the Medical Record Form. The Diet is low in sodium, and results in a natural water loss in the early stages. This – along with your weight loss – will invariably reduce blood pressure so your doctor may decide to adjust the dosage of any anti-hypertensive medication. Changes in medication must be supervised by a doctor – not by yourself or your Counsellor. If you maintain your weight loss and take regular exercise, this could be a real possibility for you.

## How will the Diet benefit my arthritis?

Arthritis is a degenerative disease affecting the weight-bearing joints. The Cambridge Diet is not a "cure", but losing excess weight helps relieve symptoms. Where attacks are triggered or aggravated by food allergies, the Cambridge Diet makes an ideal exclusion diet to follow while rogue foods are identified. A lighter body puts less strain on the joints and some patients find they need less of their anti-inflammatory drugs to alleviate the symptoms. But be careful, the joy of having less pain can make you more active, which in turn may aggravate the joints again!

## I suffer from gout. Can I still take the Diet?

Gout sufferers generally have raised blood levels of uric acid (hyperuricaemia) which can cause crystals of sodium urate to be deposited in the joints – an extremely painful condition. Using the Cambridge Diet as a Sole Source of nutrition may also raise uric acid levels, so if you are susceptible to gout, you could risk triggering an attack, particularly during the first few days of your diet. Anyone with a history of gout should be warned of this possibility and their doctor must sign the Medical Record Form and adjust their medication to prevent an attack while on 'Sole Source'

## Is the Cambridge Diet suitable for people with coeliac disease?

Yes. Coeliac disease means sufferers cannot tolerate the gluten found in wheat, oats, rye and barley. The Cambridge Diet drinks and bars are all gluten-free.

## Is the Cambridge Diet suitable for anyone with peanut allergy?

The chocolate coated bars are not suitable but all the diet drinks and soups are. The presence of peanut oil is listed in the ingredients on the wrappers of all the bars except Chocolate. Although the Chocolate flavour bar does not have peanut oil as a separate ingredient, it does contain vegetable oil, and as such there is no absolute guarantee that peanut oil may not be present even in a minute amount. Peanut allergy can be life threatening. Those that are extremely sensitive and at serious risk of anaphylactic shock if exposed to peanut in any form are extremely scrupulous about checking ingredients. A Cambridge Counsellor should be able to advise them correctly.

## Can someone with a lactose intolerance use the Cambridge Diet?

Lactose intolerance is the inability to digest lactose (milk sugar) and is caused by a deficiency of lactase – an enzyme released by the small intestine which allows milk sugar to be absorbed into the blood stream. The Cambridge Diet has a skimmed-milk base and is therefore not suitable for those with this condition. However, a small range of Cambridge Diet drinks made with soy milk is available on request. These are suitable for those who are lactose intolerant or who have a milk allergy

## Effects of the Diet

## After the second day on the Cambridge Diet I suffered a severe headache. Why is this?

Occasionally, during the initial three days a person may experience carbohydrate withdrawal and may develop a headache. This is a temporary effect and should be tolerated. A simple tablet for headaches, for example aspirin, taken for a day or two will improve the problem.

## Just after starting on the Cambridge Diet I suffered from diarrhoea. Is this normal?

This is a minor problem and is considered a possible transient effect that will last for only a short time. Some people have systems that are not used to the mineral content in the Cambridge Diet. The solutions are very simple. One is to take a bulk laxative such as Metamucil, or Fibogel. This will provide bulk to the intestinal system and alleviate the problem. Another is to consume a full glass of water following the Cambridge Diet meal in order to dilute the effect of the minerals on the body. A third solution is to take the Cambridge Diet in the form of mini meals (six half portions per day) initially to slow the mineral intake.

Another possible cause of continued diarrhoea is lactose intolerance. Some people cannot digest the lactose in milk products, and diarrhoea can occur. If this is the case, an addition of the enzyme lactase is sufficient to solve the problem. Lactase is available from chemists or health food stores and is a very inexpensive solution to the problem.

### I experience a feeling of euphoria on the Cambridge Diet. Is this normal?

This is very normal and should not cause any concern. In fact, why not just enjoy it!

### I find that I am having trouble getting my usual amount of sleep. Why is this?

It is not uncommon for a person to require less sleep when their body is put in proper nutritional balance. I know of many cases where people thought that they require 9 or 10 hours of' sleep per night, only to find that when they lost weight and maintained nutritional balance their sleep requirement dropped considerably. Having an extra hour or two awake each day may be a pleasant side effect of the Cambridge Diet.

### I feel thirsty sometimes. Is this normal?

It is normal to experience thirst on occasion when dieting. The solution is simple. Drink more liquids. At least eight glasses of liquid should be consumed each day in addition to the Cambridge Meals.

### I notice a tendency towards bad breath for the first few days. Why is this?

A mild ketosis may develop when on the Cambridge Diet as your sole source of nutrition and this may affect your breath slightly. Simply brush your teeth more often, and use mouth wash, sugar-free chewing gum or breath fresheners.

### I found shortly after starting on the Cambridge Diet that I was constipated. Is this normal?

The Cambridge Diet contains sufficient roughage for most people. When one goes on any diet including the Cambridge Diet, much less bulk is being consumed, and therefore there is much less bulk to be eliminated. As a result, bowel movements are much less frequent. This is normal, and should not cause immediate concern. When the body is ready, the bowels will move, if physical discomfort is actually being suffered then a natural laxative such as Metamucil or Fybogel should be taken according to instructions.

### Whenever I start on the Cambridge Diet plan I feel nauseated. Is this normal?

On occasion a person's body will be upset by the minerals present in the Cambridge Diet. This is usually very short lived. The benefits of the Diet far outweigh any short-term discomfort and should be tolerated. Usually, a full glass of water following your Cambridge meal will eliminate this problem. If it still persists, start taking your Cambridge Diet along with a regular meal. Another solution is to break the Cambridge Diet down into six mini meals per day, and follow each meal with a glass of water to dilute the effect of the minerals.

## I noticed that I felt dizzy a few days after starting on the Cambridge Diet.

Dizziness is a possible transient effect of any diet and should only last for a day or so. It is most often caused by the diuretic effect that accompanies any low calorie diet. During the first few days of the Diet, the body will give up a considerable amount of water, which reduces the amount of fluid circulating in the body. This can be compensated for by drinking large volumes of liquid and avoiding quick changes in position or extreme exertion during the first few days of the Diet.

## Why do I feel cold on the Cambridge Diet 'Sole Source' programme?

This is almost certainly due to a reduced thermogenic response to a reduced food intake. Large meals cause the body to generate a lot of body heat, while smaller meals produce less heat. Individuals differ widely in their thermogenic response.

For those that are affected, the cold feeling is due to the very small number of calories on the 'Sole Source' programme. Other factors that influence body heat production include the slight reduction in metabolic rate which always happens during weight loss, and of course the loss of insulating fat! Those who are sensitive to the cold need to move around more and wrap up warmly – many light layers are more effective than a single heavy layer.

## What happens to skinfolds after extensive weight loss?

After a large weight loss skin may sag. It should recover, but the speed of recovery will depend on the dieter's age, general health and level of nutrition. Ageing reduces the amount of collagen – the main support structure in the skin – making it less supple with time. Younger, rather than older skin will therefore firm up more quickly following weight loss. Massaging with lotions and oils may help. But nothing can regenerate lost collagen. It is unusual for there to be no reduction in skinfolds once weight has stabilised for a prolonged period of time, in such cases it may be necessary to eventually resort to plastic surgery. A well-balanced diet contributes greatly to good health in general and contributes to a healthy glowing skin. The complete, balanced and easily absorbed nutrition in the Cambridge Diet seems to speed up the process of firming skin and reduces skinfolds.

## Does the 'Sole Source' programme affect the menstrual cycle?

Hormone levels fluctuate when there are changes in weight – particularly in women. For most, the menstrual cycle is not affected, but some women experience increased activity and break-through bleeding may occur. Others may find that their periods stop for a while. Once target weight is reached and weight loss ceases, the metabolic rate will adjust to a new level appropriate to the new weight, and the hormones will settle down and find their own pattern again.

## I have been on the Cambridge Diet for two weeks and am getting cramp in my legs. Is the diet causing this?

A few people are prone to cramp while using the Diet as their Sole Source of nutrition. It is not caused by the diet itself, but by the increased throughput of fluid in the body's tissues. The muscle spasms result from changes in sodium levels as the water shifts between cells. The remedy for most people is to keep warm, whilst a drink of slimline tonic water just before bedtime may also help, as it contains quinine – as may "Crampex" tablets.

## I have lost 3st (42lb - 19kg) on the 'Sole Source' programme and am now experiencing some hair loss. Is this due to the Cambridge Diet?

Hair loss, with a generalised thinning of the hair, is usually linked to emotional stress, severe illness, malnutrition, hypothyroidism, hormones, and (for a few people) extensive weight loss over a sustained period of time whatever the method of weight loss used. So, it is due to a physiological response to the actual weight loss process rather than to the Diet, and the incidence is very low. Hair does re-grow, usually thicker and glossier than before. It is the "lesser of the evils" and you will have the best of both worlds – a healthy weight and a good head of hair.

*This condition should not be confused with alopecia whereby hair comes out in patches which is a medical condition needing treatment by a doctor.*

## Could the Cambridge Diet impair vision?

Very rarely, a temporary change in vision shows up if a routine eye test is performed while taking the Cambridge Diet as a Sole Source of nutrition. It can happen when the dieter is not drinking enough while taking the Diet. The lack of fluid in the body causes a loss of fluid from inside the eye, slightly affecting its shape. Drinking more fluid restores the correct shape to the eyeball. It is self-righting once 'Sole Source' is finished and does not present a problem.

## I have developed a rash: am I allergic to the Cambridge Diet?

Rashes can be caused by any number of things other than the food we eat – pollution, temperature, sunlight, fabrics, washing powders, etc. However, allergies should always be treated with great respect. Just occasionally there is something in the formula of the Cambridge Diet to which there is an allergic reaction, in which case the Diet is not suitable for that person. Stopping, then restarting the Diet is the only way to be certain if Cambridge is the cause.

## Medical Queries

## Why are women who are pregnant or breast feeding advised not to use the Cambridge Diet?

Pregnant and lactating women can use the Cambridge Diet as a nutritional supplement but not as their sole source of nutrition, because they may need more nutrients than other people.

## Will the Cambridge Diet bring on ketosis?

The Cambridge Diet is specifically formulated with 44 grams of carbohydrates in addition to the protein and fat present. This combination produces a mild ketosis which can be a benefit to those on weight-loss programmes as it gives a slight euphoric effect while somewhat curbing the appetite.

## Does the Cambridge Diet have any effect on menstrual cycle?

Rapid weight-loss with very low calorie diets may temporarily affect the menstrual cycle patterns; ovulation, however, is not interrupted. This cycle is usually corrected within a few months, as body metabolism adjusts.

## I have already had one heart attack. Can I take the Cambridge Diet?

Check with your doctor before going on any diet. The Cambridge Diet is low in cholesterol, low in sodium and low in fat. It is recommended by most heart specialists.

## *I have had surgery for cancer. Can I take the Cambridge Diet?*

There are no contra indications in using the Cambridge Diet. Scientists are looking closely at the relationship between cancer and proper nutrition, but you should check with your doctor before using the Diet.

## *Do I need my doctor's consent to use the Cambridge Diet with food?*

We would recommend that anyone wishing to follow any weight loss programme at any calorific level should check with their doctor first. All Cambridge customers need to complete a Medical Record Form whether they plan to use the Diet with or without food. Anyone on prescribed medications or with a medical condition and planning to use the Diet at less than 1500 Kcal per day should seek their doctor's consent. The same contra-indications for the 'Sole Source' programme apply to a diet of less than 1500 Kcal.

## *My doctor says I am clinically obese and that losing weight would improve my general health. I was surprised that my Counsellor insisted on my doctor signing the Medical Record Form. Is this correct?*

Your Counsellor was absolutely right. We recommend that all customers, even those in perfect health, seek their doctor's consent before starting any weight loss programme, particularly if a doctor has not been consulted during the previous 12 months. Our Counsellors are trained and are bound by a strict Code of Conduct, whereby they must insist on a doctor's signed consent before providing any product to a patient who is under medical supervision or is receiving prescribed medication. A weight in excess of Body Mass Index 30 is classified as "clinically obese" and as such is regarded as a "medical condition".

## *I have diabetes and my condition is controlled by diet. Must I see a doctor before going on the Diet?*

Yes. Nobody with diabetes should attempt to lose weight without being supervised by his or her doctor. There are two types of diabetes: insulin dependent (known as Type I) and non-insulin dependent (Type II). The Cambridge Diet is not appropriate for Type I (insulin-dependent) diabetes. Obesity may be associated with Type II diabetes. An appropriate diet, with or without medication, can help by lowering blood sugar levels. The Cambridge Diet, taken 'Sole Source', can have this beneficial effect. Because of this, the patient's medication must be discontinued at the outset and while dieting. **Only the doctor** (not the patient or the Counsellor) **can advise on this**. Once at target weight, the doctor will reassess the patient's needs. Again, adopting the maintenance programme is a good long-term health strategy.

## *What is ketosis and is it harmful?*

Ketosis is another name for the 'fat burning' process. Once the body has used up its stored carbohydrate, it then switches to using its other energy store – unwanted fat. A ketogenic diet is very low in carbohydrate. The body's stored fat is broken down into little fatty acid molecules called ketones and these circulate taking energy to all the tissues in the body. The Cambridge Diet has been carefully researched and formulated so that when used as 'Sole Source' it has just enough carbohydrate for immediate energy and none left over for storage; this induces a mild ketosis. The smallest intake of additional carbohydrate can upset this fragile balance and cause carbohydrate to be restored along with attendant water, causing a plateau or even weight gain! The mild ketosis is an intrinsic part of the design of the 'Sole Source' programme because it has significant benefits – it is the key to comfort for the dieter:

141

" It reduces the feeling of hunger – removing the temptation to err!

" It induces a sense of well-being with good energy levels

Far from being harmful, ketosis is an important safety factor – the body gets all the energy it needs from the breakdown of its fat stores, thus protecting muscle tissue and vital organs.

### What is the ketone test?

This is a simple urine test which indicates the presence of ketones. The mild ketosis induced by the Cambridge Diet ensures that sufficient ketones are produced to give adequate energy with some left over which are passed into the urine. Two simple tests are available from the chemist (and at a reduced price from Cambridge Health Plan) – Ketostix and Ketur-Test. They are plastic strips with a felt tip. The tip will react and turn pink if ketones are present in the urine. Most dieters achieve ketosis after three days on the 'Sole Source' programme. If, after this time, a test gives a negative reading (the tip does not change colour), it is reasonable to assume that the dieter is deviating from 'Sole Source' and taking in extra carbohydrate. On the other hand, a positive reading (the tip turns pink) can be very motivating for someone who is in a pre-menstrual plateau. It is tangible evidence that their body is indeed still burning off fat, even though the loss is not showing on the scales.

### What is metabolic rate and can it be damaged by rapid weight loss?

The metabolic rate represents the amount of energy the body is burning – it is the rate at which calories <u>are</u> used. Regardless of how you diet or how often, your metabolic rate is primarily determined by how much you weigh (see next question). In all methods of dieting there is an initial small reduction in metabolic rate by about 10-15%, this phase is known as 'diet mode'. It drops quickly when food is restricted and particularly on the 'Sole Source' programme, but it drops no further despite a prolonged period of further food deprivation. The metabolic rate returns to 'normal mode' when food intake returns to the appropriate amount for the actual energy expended to maintain the new weight. A lighter body will not need so many calories to move it round and will establish a metabolic rate appropriate to the new weight.

### Is Ketosis affected by someone 5'5', 15 stone taking three Cambridge Diet sachets and one bar daily?

The Cambridge Diet has been carefully researched and formulated to have an exact amount of carbohydrate. Enough for immediate energy but nothing left over for storage. The bars each contain 10g more of carbohydrate than do the drinks. Three drinks add up to 42.9 carbohydrate, four drinks 57.2g, three drinks plus a bar 67.6g! For those who are carbohydrate sensitive the latter combination could be enough to bring them out of ketosis with a consequent loss of benefits.

### Why should blood sugar levels differ some days, when intake of diet and fluids are exactly the same for someone who is Type 2 diabetic?

Even when diet and fluid intake are the same, there are other variables to take into account. In Type 2 diabetes the pancreas is still producing some insulin, though not enough for the body's needs, and production levels may vary. The body's uptake of the insulin will also be variable. Exercise increases muscle uptake of glucose and therefore reduces blood glucose levels. So the timing of the blood glucose test in relation to pancreas activity, exercise, as well as medication, the last meal and stress levels is important – these can all influence blood sugar levels.

Note: oral hypoglycaemic medication should be discounted on the 'Sole Source' programme. VLCD lowers blood sugar levels and, combined with medication, could make them go too low. The risks from blood sugar falling too low are greater than those from temporary increased blood sugar – which will automatically drop on 'Sole Source', the adjustment takes place quickly.

## I am using the 'Sole Source' programme, but have a cough and cold – what can I take?

'Sole Source' is not ideal for anyone who is below par. Also, cough and cold remedies contain carbohydrate which affects levels of ketosis and therefore the dieter's comfort. The Diet *can* be used as a nutritious part of a light diet with plenty of clear fluids for anyone who is unwell or who is convalescing. Use any over-the-counter remedy to relieve cough and cold symptoms and then, once you are fully recovered, you can restart 'Sole Source'.

## Is it all right to continue the 'Sole Source' programme if giving blood?

The 'Sole Source' programme should not be followed for one week preceding blood donation and for one week after. In fact, a centre will refuse to take blood if they know the donor is on a very low calorie diet, because blood viscosity and volume are affected by the 'Sole Source' programme.

## Product Information

## Does the Cambridge Diet contain enough protein when taken as a sole source of nutrition?

The 8½ years of research developing the Cambridge Diet concluded that 33 grams of protein per day, in combination with 44 grams of carbohydrate provide sufficient protein to maintain the lean body tissue required.

## Is Cambridge suitable for vegetarians?

There is only one item in the range which is not suitable for vegetarians – the Chicken and Mushroom Soup which contains real chicken in the flavouring. There are various degrees of vegetarianism, some stricter than others and depending upon motivation. Strict vegetarians will be reassured to know that non-animal rennet is used in the whey protein in the Cambridge meal bars. Trimmer nutrition bars however are not suitable, they contain animal rennet. Strict vegans, who shun all dairy products, will of course not be able to use either Trimmer or Cambridge Diet products, although they could use Cambridge soy products.

## Why should you not use three Cambridge Bars a day while on 'Sole Source'?

There is more carbohydrate in the bars than in the drinks and soups. Three bars in a day can contain enough carbohydrate to break the mild ketosis which you get on 'Sole Source'. Without this ketosis, you could become hungry and uncomfortable and so less likely to remain on the 'Sole Source' programme. For some people, even one bar a day can prevent ketosis. We recommend that only drinks are used during the first two weeks on the 'Sole Source' programme. A simple urine test for ketones can help with a customer who is experiencing poor weight loss on two drinks and a bar – sometimes the extra carbohydrate causes fluid retention. Some lucky individuals get into ketosis easily and can even get away with three bars a day! If your customer insists this is how they want to use the diet, make sure they drink even more water and of course monitor their ketone levels to ensure that they stay in ketosis. A warning: the complex carbohydrate in the bars can cause flatulence in some people. One a day does not usually cause a problem, three a day could be socially embarrassing!

## Weight Loss

### Will everybody lose weight on the Cambridge Diet?

Yes, the only difference is how much and how fast. Men burn more calories than women, therefore men will lose weight more quickly.

### I find that although I am faithful to my diet my weight-loss levels off from time to time. Why is this?

This is known as 'plateauing' and is very natural. Plateaus can have any number of causes. For instance, it is normal for females to plateau before menstruation, but this is fluid retention and is temporary. Often, just a little snack here and there adds enough calories to sustain the body and eliminate further weight-loss. Diet sodas generally contain a high amount of salt, and an excess of diet soda can cause plateauing.

### What weight loss can I expect?

There is a good initial weight loss in the first week on any diet. This is due to the loss of fluid which is bound up with stored carbohydrate and which the body uses for energy before tapping into its fat stores. Carbohydrate is stored in the form of glycogen in the liver, muscles, and even the fat cells of the very obese – it is like a sponge and holds four times its weight in water. On the 'Sole Source' programme there is a marked loss in the first week and the body completely exhausts its carbohydrate stores, shedding all the water that is stored with it. The Diet has been carefully formulated to contain enough carbohydrate for immediate energy but nothing left over for storage. It is not unusual to lose as much as 7lb (3½ kg) in the first week.

Once the carbohydrate store is exhausted weight loss slows down when the body switches to fat for energy. In subsequent weeks a minimum loss of about 3lb (1.5kg) can be expected. It is not unusual to lose 14lb (6kg) in the first month on the 'Sole Source' programme.

When the Cambridge Diet is used alongside food for weight loss purposes the body burns a mixture of carbohydrate and fat for energy. Some fluid is shed initially and there is usually a greater weight loss in the first week than in subsequent weeks – approx 3lb (1.5kg). An average loss of 6-8lb (3-4kg) a month can be expected on this programme.

### Why have I suddenly stopped losing weight?

Plateaux are experienced on any diet – even complete starvation! Rest assured it is always due to fluid retention and not because the diet has stopped working. Anyone following a reducing regime of 400 or 800 kcal per day would be defying the laws of nature if they did not lose weight! The body needs 800 kcal a day just to maintain body temperature at rest – that's without moving so much as a little finger! Fluid retention can be caused by any of the following:-

☐ Hormones – women can be affected before a period or during the menopause
☐ Medication – particularly hormone replacement and steroids
☐ Constipation – water is reabsorbed the longer waste products remain in the bowel
☐ Strenuous exercise – muscles tone and firm up with water
☐ Carbohydrate – water is reabsorbed with stored carbohydrate

Water is heavier and denser than fat; if fluid retention is not due to deviation from the 'Sole Source' recommendations the body will continue to burn fat for energy and though the loss is not showing on the scales it will be shown on the tape measure, and there will be a positive ketone test.

## Is it possible to 'spot' reduce?

Everyone is genetically predisposed to be a certain shape. Losing weight does not necessarily therefore result in a shape change. However, exercise may help. When combined with a weight loss programme, exercise is very beneficial for general health. Exercise does not necessarily aid weight loss – jogging a mile only burns off 100kcal – but it can give a firmer, fitter shape. Alternating between aerobic and anaerobic exercise is ideal. A fitness trainer will be able to advise regarding the latter and will recommend specific resistance exercises for each group of muscles. For aerobic exercise, simple brisk walking is ideal – or indeed any activity that increases the pulse rate, causes breathlessness and produces a little perspiration! Those who are unaccustomed to exercise should check with their doctor before starting a programme. They should start gently and gradually increase their activity level until they are doing a minimum of four thirty-minute sessions per week. The end result is a more streamlined shape with well toned muscles.

## General Nutrition

### I weigh 110 lb (50 kg) and maintain my trim figure by eating very little. I often tire easily and I wonder if I am getting proper nutrition?

Thousands of people who look trim are actually suffering from poor nutrition. They tire easily and have few energy reserves. Most of them subsist without breakfast and have very little nutritious food throughout the day. By taking the Cambridge Diet drinks three times per day along with a balanced meal, they feel altogether different. Their energy level is much higher and they are obviously in much better health.

### How can the Cambridge Diet help athletes?

It provides a very good nutritional foundation for athletes whose performance is largely dependent upon their bodies receiving the precise balance of nutrients which the Cambridge Diet provides.

### Why are prospective dieters always advised to consult their doctor before starting any weight loss programme?

There are two reasons: If it is some time since you last saw your doctor, you should have a check-up before starting a weight loss programme. Based on the results of this check-up and on your medical history, your GP can advise you on a suitable weight loss regime. Obesity can be a contributing factor in some medical conditions – for example high blood pressure (hypertension), maturity onset diabetes (diabetes Type II controlled by diet or tablets), gallbladder problems and varicose veins. It is as well, therefore, to consult your doctor before following a weight loss programme, so that your progress can be monitored and so that the dosage of your medication can be adjusted if necessary. Your doctor may recommend a Weight Care with Cambridge programme if he does not consider the 'Sole Source' programme is suitable.

### Why can some people eat 'loads' and never gain weight, while others only have to look at a cream cake to gain pounds?

Shape, weight and where we carry body fat is influenced by our genes. Of course, exercise (or lack of it), together with what and how much we eat, does have an influence. Slim people seem to eat at regular times and rarely 'snack' between meals. They tend to eat healthy, low-fat foods and, because they are carrying less weight, are more active.

## What is a calorie?

Food energy is traditionally measured in calories. One calorie is the amount of energy needed to raise the temperature of one gram of water by one degree centigrade. As the calorie is an extremely small unit, when referring to measurements of the energy value of food, the kilocalorie – equivalent to 1,000 kcal – is often used instead. Kilocalories are sometimes called Calories, with a capital C. In nutrition the larger units – kilocalories and megajoules – are used. Under the international system of units the kilocalorie has been replaced by the joule and food labels now quote energy values in first kilojoules and then kilocalories. A kilojoule = 0.238 kcal. eg. The energy value of a Chocolate Velvet Tetra Brik is 580KJ/137kcal.

# Appendices

# Appendix 1

## Composition of the Cambridge Diet

The typical contents of a Cambridge Diet sachet in the United Kingdom ...

### Macronutrients

| Ingredient | per 100ml mix | per 40g serving | per 3 servings | per 4 serving |
|---|---|---|---|---|
| Energy kJ | 219 - | 585 - | 1754 - | 2329 - |
| Energy kcal | 52 | 138 | 415 | 554 |
| Protein | 5.4 g | 14.4 g | 43.2 g | 57.6 g |
| Carbohydrate | 5.3 g | 14.1 g | 42.4 g | 56.5 g |
| of which – sugars | 4.8 g | 12.8 g | 38.4 g | 51.2 g |
| polyols | 0.0 g | 0.0 g | 0.0 g | 0.0 g |
| starch | 0.5 g | 1.3 g | 4.0 g | 5.3 g |
| Fat | 1.0 g | 2.7 g | 8.1 g | 10.8 g |
| of which – saturates | 0.2 g | 0.5 g | 1.5 g | 2.0 g |
| mono-unsaturates | 0.2 g | 0.4 g | 1.2 g | 1.7 g |
| polyunsaturates | 0.4 g | 1.1 g | 3.4 g | 4.5 g |
| cholesterol | 0.9 mg | 2.4 mg | 7.2 mg | 9.6 mg |
| Fibre | 0.9 g | 2.5 g | 7.6 g | 10.1 g |

## Micronutrients

| Ingredient | per 40g serving | | per 3 servings | | % of RDA | per 4 serving | |
|---|---|---|---|---|---|---|---|
| Sodium | 0.5 | g | 1.5 | g | | 2.0 | g |
| Vitamin A | 266.7 | µg | 800.0 | µg | 100 | 1066.7 | µg |
| Vitamin D | 1.7 | µg | 5.0 | µg | 100 | 6.6 | µg |
| Vitamin E | 3.3 | mg | 10.0 | mg | 100 | 13.3 | mg |
| Vitamin C | 20.0 | mg | 60.0 | mg | 100 | 80.0 | mg |
| Thiamin | 0.5 | mg | 1.4 | mg | 100 | 1.9 | mg |
| Riboflavin | 0.5 | mg | 1.6 | mg | 100 | 2.1 | mg |
| Niacin | 6.0 | mg | 18.0 | mg | 100 | 24.0 | mg |
| Vitamin B6 | 0.7 | mg | 2.0 | mg | 100 | 2.7 | mg |
| Folacin | 66.7 | µg | 200.0 | µg | 100 | 266.7 | µg |
| Vitamin B12 | 0.7 | µg | 2.0 | µg | 200 | 2.7 | µg |
| Biotin | 0.05 | mg | 0.15 | mg | 100 | 0.2 | mg |
| Pantothenic Acid | 2.0 | mg | 6.0 | mg | 100 | 8.0 | mg |
| Vitamin K | 40.0 | µg | 120.0 | µg | * | 160.0 | µg |
| Calcium | 304.0 | mg | 912.0 | mg | 114 | 1216.0 | mg |
| Phosphorous | 336.0 | mg | 1008.0 | mg | 126 | 1344.0 | mg |
| Iron | 4.7 | mg | 14.0 | mg | 100 | 18.6 | mg |
| Magnesium | 100.0 | mg | 300.0 | mg | 100 | 400.0 | mg |
| Zinc | 5.0 | mg | 15.0 | mg | 100 | 20.0 | mg |
| Iodine | 50.0 | µg | 150.0 | µg | 100 | 200.0 | µg |
| Potassium | 0.8 | g | 2.5 | g | * | 3.4 | g |
| Chloride | 0.7 | g | 2.0 | g | * | 2.7 | g |
| Copper | 1.0 | mg | 3.0 | mg | * | 4.0 | mg |
| Manganese | 1.3 | mg | 3.9 | mg | * | 5.2 | mg |
| Selenium | 40.0 | µg | 120.0 | µg | * | 160.0 | µg |
| Molybdenum | 80.0 | µg | 240.0 | µg | * | 320.0 | µg |
| Chromium | 40.0 | µg | 120.0 | µg | * | 160.0 | µg |

Each serving also contains 1g linoleic acid and 0.13g of linolenic acid

Each drink or soup provides at least 33% of the Recommended Daily Allowance given for vitamins and trace minerals in Council Directive 90/496/EEC

* No RDA given in Council Directive 90/496/EEC

This nutritional information will vary slightly in different countries to meet local regulations and requirements.

# *Appendix 2*

## Weight Assessment Tables

As mentioned in Chapter 1, there are a number of reliable guides to indicating whether someone is – or is not – overweight.

BMI chart     page 152
Health chart  page 153
Shape chart   page 154

# BMI Chart

The first of these is the BMI chart shown below. This allows you to look up your weight (in either metric or imperial measures) down the sides of the chart, and follow the chart horizontally until this intersects your height. The figure shown is your Body Mass Index. Remember, a figure of 20 – 25 is a normal weight range.

| | | HEIGHT | | | | | | | | | | | | | | | | | | | | | | |
|---|---|---|---|---|---|---|---|---|---|---|---|---|---|---|---|---|---|---|---|---|---|---|---|---|
| **feet** | | 4 | 4 | 4 | 5 | 5 | 5 | 5 | 5 | 5 | 5 | 5 | 5 | 5 | 5 | 5 | 6 | 6 | 6 | 6 | 6 | 6 | | |
| **ins** | | 9 | 10 | 11 | 0 | 1 | 2 | 3 | 4 | 5 | 6 | 7 | 8 | 9 | 10 | 11 | 0 | 1 | 2 | 3 | 4 | 5 | | |
| **W** | **stone** | | | | | | | | | | | | | | | | | | | | | | **kg** | **W** |
| E | 6.50 | 20 | | | | | | | | | | | | | | | | | | | | | 41.3 | E |
| I | 6.75 | 20 | 20 | | | | | | | | | | | | | | | | | | | | 42.9 | I |
| G | 7.00 | 21 | 21 | 20 | | | | | | | | | | | | | | | | | | | 44.5 | G |
| H | 7.25 | 22 | 21 | 20 | 20 | | | | | | | | | | | | | | | | | | 46.0 | H |
| T | 7.50 | 23 | 22 | 21 | 21 | 20 | | | | | | | | | | | | | | | | | 47.6 | T |
| | 7.75 | 23 | 23 | 22 | 21 | 20 | 20 | | | | | | | | | | | | | | | | 49.2 | |
| | 8.00 | 24 | 24 | 23 | 22 | 21 | 21 | 20 | | | | | | | | | | | | | | | 50.8 | |
| | 8.25 | 25 | 24 | 23 | 23 | 22 | 21 | 20 | 20 | | | | | | | | | | | | | | 52.4 | |
| | 8.50 | 26 | 25 | 24 | 23 | 22 | 22 | 21 | 20 | 20 | | | | | | | | | | | | | 54.0 | |
| | 8.75 | 26 | 26 | 25 | 24 | 23 | 23 | 22 | 21 | 20 | 20 | | | | | | | | | | | | 55.6 | |
| | 9.00 | 27 | 26 | 25 | 25 | 24 | 23 | 22 | 22 | 21 | 20 | 20 | | | | | | | | | | | 57.2 | |
| | 9.25 | 28 | 27 | 26 | 25 | 24 | 24 | 23 | 22 | 22 | 21 | 20 | 20 | | | | | | | | | | 58.7 | |
| | 9.50 | 29 | 28 | 27 | 26 | 25 | 24 | 24 | 23 | 22 | 21 | 21 | 20 | 20 | | | | | | | | | 60.3 | |
| | 9.75 | 29 | 29 | 28 | 27 | 26 | 25 | 24 | 23 | 23 | 22 | 21 | 21 | 20 | 20 | | | | | | | | 61.9 | |
| | 10.00 | 30 | 29 | 28 | 27 | 26 | 26 | 25 | 24 | 23 | 23 | 22 | 21 | 21 | 20 | 20 | | | | | | | 63.5 | |
| | 10.25 | 31 | 30 | 29 | 28 | 27 | 26 | 25 | 25 | 24 | 23 | 23 | 22 | 21 | 21 | 20 | | | | | | | 65.1 | |
| | 10.50 | 32 | 31 | 30 | 29 | 28 | 27 | 26 | 25 | 25 | 24 | 23 | 22 | 22 | 21 | 21 | 20 | | | | | | 66.7 | |
| | 10.75 | 32 | 32 | 30 | 30 | 28 | 28 | 27 | 26 | 25 | 24 | 24 | 23 | 22 | 22 | 21 | 20 | 20 | | | | | 68.3 | |
| | 11.00 | 33 | 32 | 31 | 30 | 29 | 28 | 27 | 26 | 26 | 25 | 24 | 23 | 23 | 22 | 22 | 21 | 20 | 20 | | | | 69.9 | |
| | 11.25 | 34 | 33 | 32 | 31 | 30 | 29 | 28 | 27 | 26 | 25 | 25 | 24 | 23 | 23 | 22 | 21 | 21 | 20 | 20 | | | 71.4 | |
| | 11.50 | 35 | 34 | 32 | 32 | 30 | 30 | 29 | 27 | 27 | 26 | 25 | 24 | 24 | 23 | 23 | 22 | 21 | 21 | 20 | 20 | | 73.0 | |
| | 11.75 | 35 | 35 | 33 | 32 | 31 | 30 | 29 | 28 | 27 | 26 | 26 | 25 | 24 | 24 | 23 | 22 | 22 | 21 | 21 | 20 | | 74.6 | |
| | 12.00 | | 35 | 34 | 33 | 32 | 31 | 30 | 29 | 28 | 27 | 26 | 25 | 25 | 24 | 24 | 23 | 22 | 22 | 21 | 20 | 20 | 76.2 | |
| | 12.25 | | | 35 | 34 | 32 | 32 | 30 | 29 | 29 | 28 | 27 | 26 | 25 | 25 | 24 | 23 | 23 | 22 | 22 | 21 | 20 | 77.8 | |
| | 12.50 | | | 35 | 34 | 33 | 32 | 31 | 30 | 29 | 28 | 27 | 27 | 26 | 25 | 25 | 24 | 23 | 22 | 22 | 21 | 21 | 79.4 | |
| | 12.75 | | | | 35 | 34 | 33 | 32 | 30 | 30 | 29 | 28 | 27 | 26 | 26 | 25 | 24 | 24 | 23 | 22 | 22 | 21 | 81.0 | |
| | 13.00 | | | | | 34 | 34 | 32 | 31 | 30 | 29 | 29 | 28 | 27 | 26 | 25 | 25 | 24 | 23 | 23 | 22 | 22 | 82.6 | |
| | 13.25 | | | | | 35 | 34 | 33 | 32 | 31 | 30 | 29 | 28 | 27 | 27 | 26 | 25 | 25 | 24 | 23 | 23 | 22 | 84.1 | |
| | 13.50 | | | | | | 35 | 33 | 32 | 31 | 30 | 30 | 29 | 28 | 27 | 26 | 26 | 25 | 24 | 24 | 23 | 22 | 85.7 | |
| | 13.75 | | | | | | 35 | 34 | 33 | 32 | 31 | 30 | 29 | 28 | 28 | 27 | 26 | 26 | 25 | 24 | 23 | 23 | 87.3 | |
| | 14.00 | | | | | | | 35 | 33 | 33 | 32 | 31 | 30 | 29 | 28 | 27 | 27 | 26 | 25 | 25 | 24 | 23 | 88.9 | |
| | 14.25 | | | | | | | 35 | 34 | 33 | 32 | 31 | 30 | 30 | 29 | 28 | 27 | 26 | 26 | 25 | 24 | 24 | 90.5 | |
| | 14.50 | | | | | | | | 35 | 34 | 33 | 32 | 31 | 30 | 29 | 28 | 28 | 27 | 26 | 26 | 25 | 24 | 92.1 | |
| | 14.75 | | | | | | | | 35 | 34 | 33 | 32 | 31 | 31 | 30 | 29 | 28 | 27 | 27 | 26 | 25 | 24 | 93.7 | |
| | 15.00 | | | | | | | | | 35 | 34 | 33 | 32 | 31 | 30 | 29 | 28 | 28 | 27 | 26 | 26 | 25 | 95.3 | |
| | 15.25 | | | | | | | | | | 34 | 33 | 32 | 32 | 31 | 30 | 29 | 28 | 27 | 27 | 26 | 25 | 96.8 | |
| | 15.50 | | | | | | | | | | 35 | 34 | 33 | 32 | 31 | 30 | 29 | 29 | 28 | 27 | 26 | 26 | 98.4 | |
| | 15.75 | | | | | | | | | | 35 | 35 | 33 | 33 | 32 | 31 | 30 | 29 | 28 | 28 | 27 | 26 | 100.0 | |
| | 16.00 | | | | | | | | | | | 35 | 34 | 33 | 32 | 31 | 30 | 30 | 29 | 28 | 27 | 26 | 101.6 | |
| | 16.25 | | | | | | | | | | | | 34 | 34 | 33 | 32 | 31 | 30 | 29 | 29 | 28 | 27 | 103.2 | |
| | 16.50 | | | | | | | | | | | | 35 | 34 | 33 | 32 | 31 | 31 | 30 | 29 | 28 | 27 | 104.8 | |
| | 16.75 | | | | | | | | | | | | | 35 | 34 | 33 | 32 | 31 | 30 | 29 | 29 | 28 | 106.4 | |
| | 17.00 | | | | | | | | | | | | | 35 | 34 | 33 | 32 | 32 | 31 | 30 | 29 | 28 | 108.0 | |
| | 17.25 | | | | | | | | | | | | | | 35 | 34 | 33 | 32 | 31 | 30 | 29 | 29 | 109.5 | |
| | 17.50 | | | | | | | | | | | | | | 35 | 34 | 33 | 32 | 31 | 31 | 30 | 29 | 111.1 | |
| | 17.75 | | | | | | | | | | | | | | | 35 | 34 | 33 | 32 | 31 | 30 | 29 | 112.7 | |
| | 18.00 | | | | | | | | | | | | | | | 35 | 34 | 33 | 32 | 32 | 31 | 30 | 114.3 | |
| | 18.25 | | | | | | | | | | | | | | | | 35 | 34 | 33 | 32 | 31 | 30 | 115.9 | |
| | 18.50 | | | | | | | | | | | | | | | | 35 | 34 | 33 | 33 | 32 | 31 | 117.5 | |
| | 18.75 | | | | | | | | | | | | | | | | | 35 | 34 | 33 | 32 | 31 | 119.1 | |
| | 19.00 | | | | | | | | | | | | | | | | | 35 | 34 | 33 | 32 | 31 | 120.7 | |
| | 19.25 | | | | | | | | | | | | | | | | | | 35 | 34 | 33 | 32 | 122.2 | |
| | 19.50 | | | | | | | | | | | | | | | | | | 35 | 34 | 33 | 32 | 123.8 | |
| | 19.75 | | | | | | | | | | | | | | | | | | | 35 | 34 | 33 | 125.4 | |
| | 20.00 | | | | | | | | | | | | | | | | | | | 35 | 34 | 33 | 127.0 | |
| | 20.25 | | | | | | | | | | | | | | | | | | | | 35 | 34 | 128.6 | |
| | 20.50 | | | | | | | | | | | | | | | | | | | | 35 | 34 | 130.2 | |
| | 20.75 | | | | | | | | | | | | | | | | | | | | 35 | 34 | 131.8 | |
| | 21.00 | | | | | | | | | | | | | | | | | | | | | 35 | 133.4 | |
| | 21.25 | | | | | | | | | | | | | | | | | | | | | 35 | 134.9 | |
| **mtrs** | | 1 | 1 | 1 | 1 | 1 | 1 | 1 | 1 | 1 | 1 | 1 | 1 | 1 | 1 | 1 | 1 | 1 | 1 | 1 | 1 | 1 | | |
| **HEIGHT** | | 45 | 47 | 50 | 52 | 55 | 57 | 60 | 63 | 65 | 68 | 70 | 73 | 75 | 78 | 80 | 83 | 85 | 88 | 90 | 93 | 96 | | |

## Health Risk Chart

The next chart allows you to look up your height and weight in a similar way, but is simplified into Health Risk areas.

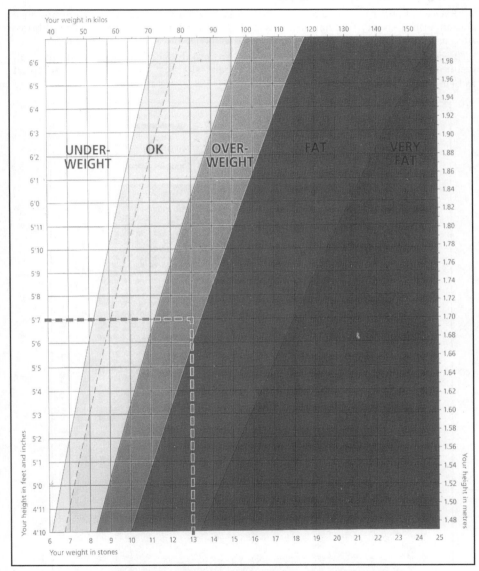

© *Health Education Authority 1999. Reproduced by permission*

## Shape Chart

The third pictorial way of assessing the risk to your health is to use the Shape Chart®, which was developed by Dr Margaret Ashwell. Her research indicated that people's health risk was also determined by the shape of their bodies, in particular, the ratio of your waist measurement to your height.

Excess fat which is stored around the stomach will give a large waist circumference and an 'apple' shape. This has been associated with risk factors for serious conditions, such as heart disease, raised blood pressure, diabetes and some types of cancer.

Excess fat which is stored under the skin, around the bottom, hips and thighs, will result in a smaller waist measurement and a 'pear' shape, which is generally accepted as being less harmful to your health.

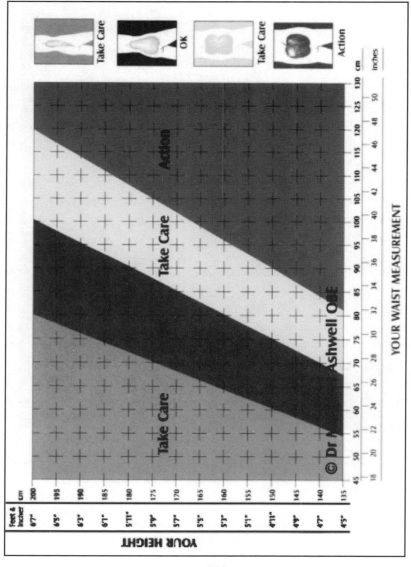

# Appendix 3

## Cambridge Contacts

As you have seen earlier in the book, Cambridge is now available in a number of countries. This list is being constantly updated and you can check changes on our website: www.cambridge-diet.com.

The contact details for Cambridge – both within the United Kingdom and around the world – are given below.

### United Kingdom

#### Cambridge Manufacturing Co Ltd

Stafford House, 10 Brakey Road, Corby, Northants, NN17 1LU
Phone:   (44) 1536 403678
Fax:   (44) 1536 401065
Web:   www.cambridge-diet.co.uk
email:   admin@cambridge-manufacturing.co.uk

#### Cambridge Export

"Grandview", North Rigton, Leeds, LS17 0DW, UK
Phone:   (44) 1423 734641
Fax:   (44) 1423 734491
web:   www.howard-foundation.com
email:   howard-foundation@netcom.co.uk

#### Cambridge Health & Weight Plan

Deben House, Old Kings Head Yard, Magdalen Street, Norwich, NR3 1JE
Phone:   (44) 1603 760777
Fax:   (44) 1603 626894
Web:   www.cambridge-diet.co.uk
email:   admin@cambridge-health-plan.co.uk

### Austria (Inc Slovenia)

#### Cambridge Diat Vertriebs Gmbh

Josef Mayburgerkai 114, A-5020 Salzburg
Phone:   (43) 662 458351
Fax:   (43) 662 458353
Web:   www.cambridge.at/
email:   cambridge@office.at

### Benelux

#### Cambridge Health Plan Benelux Bv

Postbus 2632, Gd Amersfoort
Phone:   (31) 33 4553 237
Fax:   (31) 33 4553 370
Web:   www.cambridgediet.nl
email:   info@cambridgediet.nl

### Brazil

#### Cambridge Medical Ltda

Rua Henrique Veras Do Nascimento 152 – Sala 02, Lagoa Da Conceicao, 88062-218 Florianopolis – SC, Brazil
Phone:   (55) 48 232 9414
Fax:   (55) 48 232 9414
Web:   www.dieta-cambridge.com
email:   cambridge.medical@terra.com.br

## Canada

### Natural Remedies Haven
Applewood Village Plaza, 1077 North Service Road, Unit 32, Mississauga, Ontario, L4Y 1A6
Phone:   (1) 905 306 0567
Fax:   (1) 905 272 3858
Web:
email:   weight-care@weight-care.com

## Czech Republic

### Libuse Janebova-Cambridge Diet
U Albrechtova Vrchu 11, 15500 Praha 5
Phone:   (42) 02 5162 6796
Fax:   same as above
Web:   www.cambridge-diet.cz
email:   info@cambridge-diet.cz

## Egypt

### El Marwa Trading (Cambridge Diet Egypt)
10th Of Ramadam, Cairo
Phone:   (20) 010 652 3393
Fax:
Web:
email:   krafattah@yahoo.com

## France (Inc Italy)

### Cambridge – France
16 Rue Halevy, 06000 Nice
Phone:   (33) 04 93 87 1848
Fax:   (33) 04 93 87 1759
Web:   www.cambridge-france.com
email:   Cambridge-France@wanadoo.fr

## Germany

### Nutra Products Vertirebs Gmbh
Am Wachberg 25, 50374 Erftstadt
Phone:   (49) 2235 173 68
Fax:   (49) 2235 413 130
Web:   www.cambridge-diaet.de
email:   kontakt@cambridge-diaet.de

## Hong Kong

### Personal Choice
6b, B2b Centre, 36 Connaught Road West, Sheung Wan
Phone:   (852) 2915-2066
Fax:   (852) 2975-4374
Web:   www.p-choice.com
email:   hksales@p-choice.com

## Iceland

### Cambridge Island E.H.F
Olafsbraut 19, Is-355 Olafsvik
Phone:   (35) 661 4105 or 0035 462 6620
Fax:   (35) 443 61302
Web:
email:   vaxtamotun@vaxtamotun.is

## Indonesia

### Pt Neucorindo Perkasa
ASPAC KUNINGAN, 10th Floor Suite 1008, Jl. H.R. Rasuan Said Kav X-2 No. 4, Jakarta 12950
Phone:   (62) 21 522 8555
Fax:   (62) 21 522 8366
Web:   www.neucor.co.id
email:

## Lebanon,Qatar & Kuwait

### Abyad Medical Center
Azmi Street, Abdo Center, 2nd Fl. PO Box 618, Tripoli, Lebanon
Phone:   (961) 6 443 684/5/6
Fax:   (same)
Web:
email:   aabyad@cyberia.net.lb

## Malaysia/Brunei

### Neucor Alliance (M) Sdn Bhd
No 253-257 Jalan Perkasa Satu, Taman Maluri, Cheras, 55100 Kuala Lumpur
Phone:   (60) 3 9281 3760
Fax:   (60) 3 9281 4776
Web:   www.neucor.com.my
email:   weilian@neucor.com.my

## Malta

### Estetika Co Ltd
Shamrock House, Dingli Street, Sliema, Slm 09
Phone:   (356) 2133 8265/2363
Fax:     (356) 2134 0388
Web:    www.estetika.com.mt
email:   office@estetika.com.mt

## Mauritius

### Smith Naturals Co Ltd
Newry Complex, 85 St Jean Street, Quatre Bornes
Phone:   (230) 464 2019/454 3422
Fax:     (230) 464 1298
Web:
email:   dr.siddick@smithnat.com

## Mexico

### Medlife
General Sostenes Rocha No. 57, Col. Ampl. Daniel Garza, C.P. 11870, Mexico City
Phone:   (52) 55-52-71-5576 or (52) 55-52-71-6697
Fax:     (52) 55-261-46937
Web:
email:   medlife@prodigy.net.mx

## Norway

### Midelfart & Co A/S
Ringeriksveien 16, Po Box 644, 3412 Lierstranda
Phone:   (47) 32 85 71 00
Fax:     (47) 32 85 71 90/91
Web:    www.cambridgekuren.no;
          www.midelfart.no
email:   peter.carlsson@midelfart.no

## Oman

### Mrs Rachel Dacruz
PO Box 437, Postal Code 133, Al Khuwair, Muscat
Phone:   (968) 942 0062
Fax:
Web:
email:   babe_rachel1@hotmail.com

## Philippines

### Personal Touch
Unit 2, 75 East Capitol Drive, Bo. Kapitolyo, 1603 Pasig City
Phone:   (632) 687 7227
Fax:     (632) 747 9218
Web:    www.p-choice.com
email:   rpsales@p-choice.com

## Poland

### Hol-Trade Ltd (S.P. Zoo)
Belgradzka 4, 02793 Warsaw
Phone:   (48) 22 859 03 04
Fax:     (Same)
Web:
email:   biuro@dieta-cambridge.pl

## Singapore

### Neucor Holdings Pte Ltd
No 10, Upper Aljunied Link #06-02, York International Industrial Bldg, 367904
Phone:   (65) 6280 1169
Fax:     (65) 6285 4515
Web:    www.thecambridgediet.com
email:   louisa@neucor.com

## Sweden (Inc Denmark & Finland)

### Cambridge Kuren Sverige Ab

Eliegaton 20, 17273 Sundbyberg
Phone:   (46) 8 730 02 01
Fax:      (46) 8 83 41 81
Web:     www.cambridgekuren.se
email:   cambridgekuren@swipnet.se

## Switzerland

### Ifrec SA RL,

Case Postale 67, Ch-1610 Oron La Ville
Phone:   (41) 79 212 0360
Fax:      (41) 21 907 9091
Web:     www.ifrec-sarl.ch
email:   ifrec@ifrec-sarl.ch

## Taiwan

### Trustwell Trading Co Ltd

5th Fl, 381 FU HSING S Rd, Sec 2, Taipei
Phone:   (886) 2 2733 2297
Fax:      (886) 2 2735 4291/2733/6201
Web:     www.trustwell.com.mt
email:   trust@trustwell.com.tw

## Thailand

### Alex Health Products Co Ltd

Laksi Square, 688/28-30 Changwatana Road,
Bangkhen, Bangkok 10220
Phone:   (66) 252 16 100
Fax:      (66) 252 16 099
Web:
email:

## Turkey

### Mrs Nilgun Okmen

Seher Yildizi Sk. 28/6, 80630 Etiler-Istanbul
Phone:   (90) 212-257-9138
Fax:      (90) 212-257-4149
Web:
email:   nilgunokmen@hotmail.com

## United States

### ("Dr Howard's Success") Immediate Rewards Inc

11631 Belleville Road, Belleville, Mi 48111
Phone:   (1) 734 699 8470
Fax:      (1) 734 699 5053 or 697 5050
Web:     www.successdiet.com
email:   succesdiet@aol.com

# App 4

# Bibliography

## Books on the Cambridge Diet

Birch,RD; 'The Cambridge Diet. Medically speaking'; 1982, Hexi Publishing

Blanton B, Coldstein JM, Silverman A; *'The Cambridge Diet Psychologically Speaking'*, 1983, Breakthrough Publishing

Boe E; *'The Official Cambridge Diet Book'*; 1983. Bantam Books, New York.

Ignasias S & Dennis; *'Recipes for use with the internationally acclaimed Cambridge Diet Plan'*; 1983, SIim-Lines Publications

Kreitzman SN & Howard AN; *'The Swansea Trial: Body composition and metabolic studies with a VLCD'*; 1993; Smith Gordon

Marks J & Howard AN; *'The Cambridge Diet: A Manual for Practitioners'*; 1997; Cambridge Export Limited

Wilson FC; *'The Cambridge Miracle'*;1983, Atlantis Publishing

## Other Books

Blackburn GL & Bray GA. (Editors), *'Management of Obesity by Severe Calorie Restriction'*; PSG Publishing

Costain L; *'Diet Trials: How to Succeed at Dieting'*; 2003, BBC Publicatioins

Critser G; *'Fat Land - How Americans became the fattest people in the world'*; 2003, Penguin

Dunkeld, J; *'The Good Diet Guide'*; 1995, Robinson Publishing

Kuntzleman CT & the Editors of Consumer Guide; *'The Complete Book of Exercise'*; 1979, GK Hall

Walford RL; *'Maximum Life Span'*; 1983, WW Norton

## Articles

Andersen T, Backer OG, Astrup A & Quaade F; 'Horizontal or vertical banded gastroplasty after treatment with very low calorie formula diet: a randomised trial' International Journ of Obesity, 11: 295-304, 1987.

Anderson, Konz, Frederich & Wood; 'Long-term weight loss maintenance: a meta analysis of US studies'; Am Soc of Clin Nutrition, 2001

Ashwell MA, Cole TJ & Dixon AK; 'Ratio of waist circumference to height is strong predictor of intra-abdominal fat'; British Medical Journal, 313: 559-560, 1996.

Astrup A, Rossner S; 'Lessons from Obesity Management Programmes: Greater Initial Weight Loss Improves Long-term Maintenance'; Obesity Reviews, 2000

Ayyad C, Andersen T; 'Long-term Efficacy of Dietary Treatment of Obesity: A systematic Review of Studies published between 1931 and 1999'; Obesity Reviews, 2000.

Beeson V, Ray C, Coxon A & Kreitzman S; 'The myth of the yo-yo: Consistent rate of weight loss with successive dieting by VLCD'; International Journ of Obesity, 13: suppl 2, 135-139, 1989.

Bray GA; 'Complications of obesity'; Ann IM, 103; 1052-1062, 1985.

Capstick F et al; 'VLCD: a useful alternative in the treatment of the obese NIDDM patient'; Diabetes Res Clin Pract 1996; 36, 105-11

Cook RF, Howard AN, & Mills IH, 'Low-dose mianserin as adjuvant therapy in obese patients treated by a very low calorie diet', International Journal of Obesity, 5, 1981, pp. 267-72.

Coxon A, Kreitzman SN, Howard AN, Morgan WD, Johnson P, Compston JE & Eston R; 'Change in body compositon and energy balance on VLCD: a multicentre study'; Am Jorn of Clin Nutrition, 56: suppl 1, 303, 1992.

Department of Health; 'The Health of the Nation: a strategy for health in England'; HMSO, London, 1992

Department of Health & Social Security; Report on Health and Social Subjects No 31: 'The use of very low calorie diets in obesity'; HMSO, London, 1987

DiBiase G, Mattioli PL, Contaldo F & Mancini M; 'A very low calorie formula diet (Cambridge Diet) for the treatment of diabetic-obese patients'; International Journ of Obesity, 5: 319-324, 1981.

Grant AM, Edwards OM, Howard AN, Challand G, Wraight EP & Mills IH, 'Thyroidal hormone metabolism in obesity during semi-starvation', Clinical Endocrinology, 9, 1978, pp. 227-31

Henry RR, Wallace P & Olefsky CM; 'The effects of weight loss on the mechanisms of hyperglycemia in obese non-insulin-dependent diabetes mellitus'; Diabetes, 35: 990-997. 1986a.

Henry RR, Wiest-Kent TA, Scheaffer L, Kolterman, OG, & Olefsky JM; 'Metabolic consequences of VLCD therapy in obese non-insulin-dependent and non-diabetic subjects'; Diabetes, 35: 155-164, 1986b.

Hickey N, Daly L, Bourke G & Mulcahy R; 'Out-patient treatment of obesity with a very low calorie formula diet'; International Journ of Obesity, 5: 227-230, 1981.

Howard AN & McLean Baird I; 'A long-term evaluation of very low calorie semi-synthetic diets: an inpatient/outpatient study with egg albumin as the protein source', International Journal of Obesity, 1, 1977, pp. 63-78.

Howard AN & McLean Baird I; 'Physiopathology of protein metabolism in relation to very low calorie regimens', in Recent Advances in Obesity Research: III, 1981,John Libbey & Co., London.

Howard AN & McLean Baird I; 'The treatment of obesity by low calorie semi-synthetic diets', in Recent Advances in Obesity Research: 1., edited by Howard A.N., 1974, Newman Publishing, pp. 270-3.

Howard AN & McLean Baird I; 'Very low calorie semi-synthetic diets in the treatment of obesity. An inpatient/outpatient study', Nutr. Metab., 21, 1977, pp. 59-61.

Howard AN & McLean Baird I; 'A long-term evaluation of very low calorie semi-synthetic diets: an inpatient/out patient study with egg albumen as the protein source'; International Journ of Obesity, 1: 63-78, 1977.

Howard AN & McLean Baird I; 'The treatment of obesity by low calorie semi-synthetic diets'; In: Recent Advances in Obesity Research. No. 1, AN Howard (ed), Newman Publishing Ltd., 270-273, 1974.

Howard AN, Grant A, Challand G, Wraight E.P & Edwards 0; 'Thyroid metabolism in obese subjects after a very low calorie diet', 1977, Second International Congress on Obesity.

Howard AN, Grant A, Challand G, Wraight E.P & Edwards 0; 'Thyroid metabolism in obese subjects after a very low calorie diet', International Journal of Obesity, 2, 1978, p. 391.

160

Howard AN, Grant A, Edwards 0, Littlewood ER & McLean Baird I; 'The treatment of obesity with a very low calorie liquid formula diet: an inpatient! outpatient comparison using skimmed milk protein as the chief protein source', International Journal of Obesity, 2, 1978, pp. 321-32.

Howard AN, Grant A, Edwards O, Littlewood ER & McLean Baird I; 'The treatment of obesity with a very low calorie liquid formula diet: an inpatient/out-patient comparison using skimmed milk protein as the chief protein source'; International Journ of Obesity, 2: 321-332 1978.

Howard AN; 'Dietary treatment of obesity', in Obesity. Its Pathogenesis and Management, edited by Silverstone, T., 1975, Medical and Technical Publishing Co., pp.123-54.

Howard AN; 'The Cambridge Diet: A response to criticism',]. Obesity and Weight Regulation, 3, 1984, pp.65-84.

Howard AN; 'The historical development, efficacy and safety of very low calorie diets', International Journal of Obesity, 5, 1981, pp. 195-208.

Howard AN; 'The treatment of obesity by starvation and semi-starvation', in The Treatment of Obesity, edited by Munro, J.F., 1979, MTP Press, pp. 139-64

Howard AN; 'The historical development, efficacy and safety of VLCDs'; International Journ of Obesity, 5: 195-208, 1981.

Howard AN; 'The Swansea trial: its purpose and rationale'; IN: 'The Swansea Trials', pp 15-23, 1993 (see Books above).

James WPT, Davies HI, Bailes J & Dauncey MJ; 'Elevated metabolic rates in obesity'; Lancet, 1: 1122-1125, 1978.

Jebb SA et al; 'No evidence of excessive losses of protein during acute weight loss'; MRC Dunn Clin Nutrition Centre poster presented at 8th International Congress on Obesity, Paris 1998

Jebb SA & Goldberg GR; 'Efficacy of very low-energy diets and meal replacements in the treatment of obesity'; J Hum Nut & Diet, 11, 219-225, 1998.

Kirschner MA et al; 'An 8-year experience with a very low calorie formula diet for control of major obesity'; Obesity Research 9, Nov 2001, Supp 4

Kreitzman S, Coxon, A. Johnson P & Morgan W; 'Dependence of weight loss during VLCD on total energy expenditure rather than resting metabolic rate associated with fat free mass'; Am Jorn of Clin Nutrition, 56: suppl 1, 258-261, 1992.

Kreitzman S; Factors influencing body composition during VLCDs; Am Jorn of Clin Nutrition, 56: suppl 1, 217-223, 1992.

Kreitzman SN & Coxon A; Independence of body composition from mode, rate or direction of weight change in women as a result of dieting or regaining weight; International Journ of Obesity, 14: 904, 1990.

Kreitzman, S.N., Pedersen, M., Budell, W., Nichols, D., Krissman, P. and Clements, M., 'Safety and Effectiveness of Weight Reduction Using a Very Low Calorie Formulated Food', Arch. Intern. Med., 144, 1984, pp.747-50.

Krotkiewski M, Toss L, Bjorntorp P & Holm G; 'The effect of a very low calorie diet with and without chronic exercise on thyroid and sex hormones, plasma proteins, oxygen uptake, insulin and c peptide concentrations in obese women', International Journal of Obesity, 5, 1981, pp. 287-93.

Lamberts SWJ, Visser TJ, & Wilson JHP; 'The influence of caloric restrictions on serum prolactin', International Journal of Obesity, 3, 1979, pp. 75-81.

McLean Baird I., & Howard AN; 'A double blind trial of mazindol using a very low calorie formula diet', International Journal of Obesity, 1, 1977, pp. 271-8.

McLean Baird I; 'Low calorie formula diets – are they safe?' International Journal of Obesity, k5 1981, pp.249-56.

McLean Baird I, Littlewood ER & Howard AN, 'Safety of very low calorie diets', International Journal of Obesity, 3, 1979, 399.

McLean Baird I, Parsons, R.L. and Howard, A.N., 'Clinical and metabolic studies of chemically defined diets in the management of obesity', Metabolism, 23, 1974, pp. 645-57.

Moore R, Grant AM, Howard AN & Mills IH; 'Treatment of Obesity with triiodothyronine and a very low calorie liquid formula diet', The Lancet, Feb. 2, 1980, pp. 223-6.

Moore R, Grant AM, Howard AN, Mehrishi JN, & Mills IH; 'Changes in thyroid hormone levels, kinetics and cell receptors in obese patients treated with $T_3$ and a very low calorie formula diet', in Recent Advances in Clinical Nutrition, 1981,J. Libbey & Co., London.

Moore R, Mehrishi JN, Verdoorn C & Mills IH, 'The role of $T_3$ and its receptor in efficient metabolisers receiving very low calorie diets', International Journal of Obesity 5, 1981, pp. 283-96.

Mustajoki P, Pekkarinen T; 'Very Low Energy Diets in the Treatment of Obesity'; Obesity Reviews, 2001

Paisley P B  et al; An intensive weight loss programme for obese Type II diabetics – 1 year results; Abstract for European Obesity Society September 1996.

Pekkarinen T, Takala I, & Mustajoki P; Weight loss with very-low-calorie diet and cardiovascular risk factors in moderately obese women: One-year follow-up study including ambulatory blood pressure monitoring; International Journ of Obesity, (1998) 22, 661-666.

Pekkarinen & & Mustajoki P; 'Use iof Very Low Calorie Diet in preoperative weight loss: efficacy and safety; Obesity Research 1997

Quaade F, & Astrup A; Initial VLCD improves ultimate weight loss; International Journ of Obesity, 13: suppl, 107-111, 1989.

Rattan S, Coxon A, Kreitzman S & Lemons A; Maintenance of weight loss with recovery of resting metabolic rate following 8 weeks of very low calorie dieting; International Journ of Obesity, 13: suppl 2, 189-192, 1989.

Ryde SJ, Morgan WD, Birks JL, Dutton J; Changes in body composition following a VLCD; Basic Life Sci, 60: 263-265, 1993a.

Ryttig KP & Rossner S; 'Weight maintenance after a VLCD weight period and the effects of VLCD supplementation'; Journ Int'l Medicine 236; pp233-9; 1995

Ryttig KP, Flaten H & Rossner S; 'Long-term effects of a VLCD (Nutrilett) in obesity treatment. A prospective, randomised, comparison between VLCD and hypocaloric diet+behaviour modification and their combination'; Int'l Journ of Obesity,  (1997) 21: 574-579.

Saris WHM; 'Very Low Calorie Diets and sustained weight loss'; Obesity Research 9; Supp4, Nov 2001

Scott BC, Beeson V and Kreitzman SN; VLCD: a potential first line in treatment for obese hypertensives; Clin Sci, 92: 2, 1997.

Shapiro H, Weinkove C, Coxon A, Kreitzman S & Rodgers M; Three year hospital experience with control of major obesity by VLCD in medically compromised individuals; International Journ of Obesity, 13: suppl 2, 125-129, 1989.

Shapiro, H.J., 'Report of a comparative study: a new very low calorie formula diet versus a conventional diet in the treatment of obesity', International Journal of Obesity, 2, 1978, p. 392.

Simonen P, Gylling H, Howard AN & Miettinen TA; 'Introducing a new component of the metabloic syndrome: low cholesterol absorption'; Amer Journ Clin Nutrition; 72:82-8, 2000

Trott, DC and Tyler, FH; Evaluation of the Cambridge Diet. A New Very Low Calorie Liquid Formula Diet; Western Journal of Medicine, 30, no. 1, 1981, pp. 18-20.

Wilson JHP & Lamberts SWJ; Nitrogen balance in obese patients receiving a very low calorie liquid formula diet; American Journal of Clinical Nutrition, 32, 1979, pp. 1612-16.

Wilson JHP & Lamberts SWJ; The effect of triiodothyronine on weight-loss and nitrogen balance of obese patients on a very low calorie liquid formula diet; International Journal of Obesity, 5, 1981, pp. 279-82.

Wilson JHP & Lamberts SWJ; The effect of obesity and drastic caloric restriction on serum prolactin and thyroid stimulating hormone; International Journal of Obesity, 5, 1981, pp. 275-8